Praise for *Confessions of a Trauma Junkie*

"A must read for those who choose to subject themselves to life at its best and at its worst. Sherry offers insight in the Emergency Response business that most people cannot imagine. This book details life through the eyes of a caring individual who is a devoted CISM practitioner and true professional, who continually accepts the crisis presented, employs best practices, focuses on the mission, and makes the trauma, pain and suffering a little easier to manage."

—Maj Gen Richard L. Bowling,
former Commanding General, USAF Auxiliary (CAP)

"We are not alone. Sherry Mayo shares experiences and unique personal insights of first responders. Told with poetry, sensitivity and a touch of humor at times, all are real, providing views into realities EMTs, Nurses, and other first responders encounter. Emotions shared bind this fraternity/sorority together in understanding, service and goals. Recommended reading for anyone working with trauma, crises, critical incidents in any profession. It's heartening to know we share such common experiences and support from our peers."

—George W. Doherty, MS, LPC, President
Rocky Mountain Region Disaster Mental Health Institute

"In this book, Sherry has captured the essence of working with people who have witnessed trauma. It made me cry, it made me laugh, it helped me to understand differently the work of our Emergency Services Personnel. I consider this a 'MUST READ' for all of us who wish to be helpful to those who work in these professions."

— Dennis Potter, LMSW, CAAC, FAAETS, ICISF Instructor

"Sherry has encapsulated the first responder human lifestyle and given it soul. Makes you appreciate those who serve others in what happens in the streets of America every day. Sherry gracefully exposes the dreaded 'F' word...*Feelings*... and will absolutely touch every reader in surprising ways."

—Police Officer (Ret.) Pete Volkmann, MSW, EMT
Ossining, NY Police Department

Confessions of a Trauma Junkie

My Life as a Nurse Paramedic
Second Edition

Sherry Lynn Jones, EdD, MS, RN, FAAETS

Reflections of America Series

From Modern History Press

Ann Arbor, Michigan

Library of Congress Cataloging-in-Publication Data

Mayo, Sherry Jones, 1955-
 Confessions of a trauma junkie : my life as a nurse paramedic / by Sherry Jones Mayo.
    p. ; cm. -- (Reflections of America series)
 Includes bibliographical references and index.
 ISBN-13: 978-1-61599-341-3 (trade paper : alk. paper)
 ISBN-13: 978-1-61599-342-0 (hardcover : alk. paper)
 1. Mayo, Sherry Jones, 1955- 2. Nurses--Biography. 3. Emergency medical technicians--Biography. 4. Emergency nursing--Biography. I. Title. II. Series: Reflections of America series.
 [DNLM: 1. Mayo, Sherry Jones, 1955- 2. Emergency Medical Technicians--Personal Narratives. 3. Nurses--Personal Narratives. 4. Emergency Medical Services--Personal Narratives. 5. Emergency Nursing--Personal Narratives. WZ 100 M47315 2009]
 RT120.E4M345 2009
 610.73092--dc22
                    2009017672

Distributed by Ingram Book Group (USA/CAN), Bertram's Books (UK/EU)

Published by Modern History Press,
www.ModernHistoryPress.com

An Imprint of Loving Healing Press
5145 Pontiac Trail
Ann Arbor, MI 48105
www.LHPress.com
info@LovingHealing.com
Toll free 888-761-6268
Fax 734-663-6681

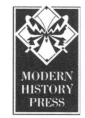

To Sean Kovacs and Andrew Campbell,
kind and caring grandsons who help me
to live graciously and mindfully.

With Love, from Nona

Contents

Foreword

Writing a foreword for *Confessions of a Trauma Junkie* is a true honor. As someone who has the privilege of knowing Sherry Lynn Jones, it is a chance to express admiration and respect. Her writing conveys the essence of what it means to be a professional. What certainly distinguishes this book is her ability also to show us the human side of the helping professions she has practiced. The emotional rewards and challenges of helping those in crisis are shown to us the way they are lived…with passion, humility, intensity, and sometimes, painfully. Sherry shows us what those outside of these professions may never see… the joys, pains, and privileges that come from working with those in crisis. This is a powerful, honest, and moving account of an amazing career.

Having had the privilege of knowing Sherry throughout her career, I am reminded how deeply the call to service to others can live inside someone. Both through her direct patient care, and her service to other professionals as a crisis responder, and her teaching Sherry embodies what it means to be professional, caring, compassionate, and hilarious. The humor that helps us all cope and serves as such a source of resilience is a wonderful side of this story. The crisis intervention field focuses much of our work on promoting resilience in the face of trauma. Sherry gives us a beautiful first person account of how it works, and how the way we care for people matters in the worst moments of their lives.

This book, much like its author, is inspirational. Readers will come away wiser, and more respectful of the work of crisis professionals. Sherry's dedication to the people she serves, her dedication to continually learning and growing, and her dynamic presence come alive as you read the stories she so artfully tells us. Be prepared to be impacted!

Victor Welzant, Psy.D.
Director of Education and Training, ICISF

Preface: The Healer Within

If we accept the premise that each of us is a special creation placed on Earth to perform as well as our design would enable us, I believe there is an individual choice whether to act upon inherent capabilities and gifts. In this case and this book, this reference points to the healer within. I believe that all the *secrets* held since the beginnings of time are for each of us to explore. No special dispensation is necessary; we have access to it all and the capability to understand and take action. We have permission to enter into a world of limitless possibility. We truly choose our own adventures.

Sometimes the search for (and development of) talents takes one on diverse paths of self-discovery. I hold in memory a crystal image of my day of realization, etched with full-spectrum coloration when the dark curtain of ignorance fell away, and the door to answers flew open. That moment prompted exploration into the mind/body connection where psychology and medicine merge. I am still wading in that pool, taking it all in, and learning as I go along. While learning, I laugh a lot because lunacy abounds, and I sometimes cry because humanity suffers so much pain. In that place between lunacy and sorrow, I grab a homemade water pistol (30cc syringe with a 22-gauge plastic IV catheter) and take aim.

This book is a peek into the world of EMS, ER, and corrections folks from those who do those jobs daily. It is comprised of essays and quotes—all true though sometimes compiled—from EMTs, corrections folks, and RNs around the country (names and some details occasionally changed to protect the guilty). This is your opportunity to share in the pain and laughter (not just the patient's, but also our own) while we go through life trying to keep from succumbing to whatever evil presents itself. We fight the enemy (death) with everything we have and try to keep a sense of humor while doing it. There are many more stories; these are a handful written by a Paramedic-RN, who has worked rural, country and city EMS as well as an urban trauma center since 1989. In the years following the first *Confessions*, I worked in an inpatient psychiatric nurse in a state corrections facility. Please do not take offense—some of the items shared are less than politically correct.

Walk a mile in our shoes and we will talk about what truly offends. Walk two miles and you'll have stories of your own and a greater understanding of the sights, smells, and experiences of those who expertly do what nobody should ever have to do.

How we have separated the mind from the body baffles me. We know that our cells have an innate intelligence and somehow group with other cells that hold a common desire to sustain growth and continue life. Similar cells combine to develop tissues; related tissues become organs, systems form and the infinitely small parts together become a functional whole. Our bodies are composed of energy and information. There is intelligence in each of the cells as there is intelligence in the organism (human being), directing and guiding toward the collective good and development of the entity.

By the end of one year, 98% of the body's atoms exchange for new ones, a built-in mechanism for change, renewal, and regeneration. Unifying the body and mind toward positive and forward growth is sometimes a challenge when one stumbles over pebbles (or boulders) in their paths. Balance is interrupted, and intervention is necessary (from internal or external sources) to recover physical, mental, and emotional balance.

What we do not know is what happens at that moment between thoughts, the moment between desiring and directing a physical action and its ultimate implementation. When we discover mysteries of the mind, we continue to tread water in their interpretations. Despite intellect, education, desire, and experience, how we communicate is a mystery, too, as any married couple will tell you.

Life is a journey of discovery. Learning is a relatively permanent transformation in an organism resultant of experience or acquired information. Working in the world of medicine (and mental health) provides multitudes of opportunity for education and change. I am emphatically not the person I was before working the streets, the ER, the psych ward, or the state prison. I could not have known where searching for answers to the pain I witnessed in others as well as myself would lead.

A gateway opened, and I have stepped across a threshold to a new plane of existence that in the past appeared only fleetingly in the back of my consciousness. I am not a creature who can trek through life loving selectively and denying my affiliation with humanity or the universe. We are connected. I am a spiritual being encased in a physical body, over which I have tremendous influence despite my immature denial in years past, who maintains a conscious walk into self and cosmic awareness.

The quest for answers and direction in response to emotional pain also led me to Jeffrey T. Mitchell, Ph.D., C.T.S.; George S, Everly, Jr., Ph.D., ABPP; Dennis Potter, LMSW, CAAC, FAAETS; Don Howell, former ICISF executive director at ICISF; and my dear friend and mentor, Victor Welzant, PsyD, all from the International Critical Incident Stress Foundation (ICISF). They have provided a program of interventions that I have used and seen successfully applied countless times to thousands of people. I thank these brilliant and caring leaders for their unwavering guidance as I continue to learn from them.

From my family, of course, I have learned the most. From my children, I have come to know and appreciate (and hopefully apply) unconditional love. They have gone from being my students to showing me wonderment I could not have imagined, and I continue to learn from them daily.

"Topher," my sweet and generous computer genius son (programming at age six) has always had a vision that others could not see or understand. Still, he patiently points toward those unseen things that are beyond common comprehension, good-naturedly teaching concepts from the complex to the simple, like an introduction to the Mandelbrot set or showing me how to build and maintain a fire. Sometimes the mother but certainly always the devoted daughter and comedian, Michele Denise (named after her Grandfather Michael Dennis, and married to firefighter-medic Scott) lovingly keeps me from embarrassing myself in public (sometimes), attempts to influence my wardrobe and shows me how not to grow up. Grandson Sean is the new Topher, his and Angie's son, who looks at me with the eyes of a very old soul as did his father. Grandson Andrew teaches me mindfulness and reminds me how to have fun and love unconditionally.

My sweet Italian Mama, who always believed in her children regardless of obstacles, taught us that anything was possible. You just have to find the way, and there is *always* a way. Dad was a Marine, who gave me a strong sense of patriotism, which translated into community service, an idea of giving back, that through giving I receive so much more than I could ever give. Sister Nonie, who is my second mama and also a writer, educated me in the ways of Suzy Homemaker and how (eventually) to stand up for any living creature in need, including myself. Most of us have someone in our lives to offer love and caring, even if our support systems are animals (like my furry children, Izzy and Ziva). Our supports offer friendship, love, a sense of presence in times of need, and refill our emotional tanks when those reserves threaten to run dry. They hold us up and sustain us when we cannot walk alone.

For all the EMTs, firefighters and police who have or are still working the road, you are my heroes. You are doing the best job that I have ever loved, and I pray for you often. You are my family, and we share an inexplicable and unbreakable bond, even if we have never met..

Emergency Room staff, you and I stand together to bear the lunacy and sorrow, to fight our enemies (death, injury, and illness) while trying to educate people and keep a sense of humor (as well as some level of empathy) intact. Keep your 16 gauge needles handy, remember the value of a B-52, and never, ever turn your back on a patient, however cooperative they were just a moment before.

To my corrections peeps, few will understand. Keep your heads about you, hearts open, and know that the good you do, though often unrecognized, reflects in The World. Remember that there are human souls within that underbelly of society, and you *can* save some.

Keep your chins up, chests out, and remember that you do the impossible every day, in numbers no one could imagine, at a speed that rivals Olympic champions. Keep up the good fight, my brothers and sisters. We need to nurture that bond between us because no one, however much they see or read or witness, understands what we do. It is our private world, and this book will let outside folks see a little more of what we are made of and how we do the impossible every day, how we triumph when there is sometimes no clear winner.

Most of all please continue to love what you do. If you do not have the same passion you started with, consider finding another avenue in which to channel your energies. For your sake, and that of your families, you need to keep your soul and your sanity intact.

There are many stories and references in this book about Marson. He is one in my holy trinity of mentors: Ma, Wheaton, and Benson. I love and respect all three. I asked Dr. Wheaton to write a few words acknowledging Dr. Ma, and what Doug gave me is in true, no-nonsense, tell-it-like-it-is ER doc style. This is how we roll.

In Memoriam: Marson Ma Jr. MD
February 23, 1955 - June 14, 2015

Writing an acknowledgment is too emotional, and Marson hated that stuff at the end, the last year of his life. He bled to death on a weekly basis. I have no idea how many units of packed cells that guy got in that year with the chemo and the bullshit of the whole thing. Pancreatic cancer with liver metastasis and an intestinal luminal bleeding mass, a mass so dysplastic that the pathology specimen sent to U of M, and on to MD Anderson, could not be typed. I mean come on, get your affairs in order; the dirt nap is coming.

Mila, his wife, told me that Marson was showing Milson, his son, how to winterize the sprinkler system last fall. Marson goes out in the back yard after showing Milson the control box, and he is so weak and tired he vagals out and collapses. He is on the ground, turns his head, and screams, "Fire, Zone 3!" That was the man. That is a man.

The best times I had with him towards the end were when the chemo started to gain some ground and Mila, Marson, and I would go to the Coney Island on Gratiot and I-696. I could get him to drink a strawberry shake. Sunny autumn day, Marson was almost like himself, funny and joking around, yet both of us knew it would not last. Many things I could say, but nothing covers it. Death solves everything and nothing, you know. Marson was prolific as a doctor, as a worker; he saw 183,000 patients in 23 years of practice, most of them at a Level I trauma center or worse... like someplace with no backup. A role model to me, and any doctor, resident or otherwise, that he ever worked with. I was a year behind Marson in training, and like a little brother to him. I was the first resident Marson ever trained.

—Douglas Wheaton, MD

Preface to the 2nd Edition

Medics and nurses continually learn and evolve personally and in practice. Beyond the boots-on-the-ground street views and feet-to-the-fire hospital views, I found something new. Corrections. Meeting trauma, psych, and nursing needs of high-security prison populations is intense. Not judging is imperative, remaining neutral in a community where inmates sometimes run the asylum. With the primary goal of going home each day, alive and uninjured, corrections nurses up the ante of awareness, employ tough yet tender no-nonsense attitudes, and rely on Corrections Officers for their safety. This edition updates previously told stories, shares new experiences, provides more mature perceptions, and peeks into the survival humor of state prison staff.

First edition readers were kind enough to give feedback. Thank you; I listened. This version represents a major overhaul based on your constructive criticisms and includes updated outcomes. New knowledge includes strongly and preemptively educating about resilience and coping skills. "Nurses Occupational Trauma Exposure, Resilience, and Coping Education" is my dissertation (Google it) and swan song for all who brave the tough stuff to care for others. We are not alone.

<table>
<tr><td>

1

</td><td>

On the Road Again
Stories from
Emergency Services Workers

</td></tr>
</table>

When least expected, an Emergency Services (ES) worker might get the call that will change his life. Critical Incident Stress Management (CISM) is the standard of care in handling these emotionally traumatic circumstances and experiences, but CISM is not practiced or appropriately applied everywhere. Some folks are emotionally lost after a call so soul-stirring they cannot mentally escape. The worker can become a secondary victim of trauma. No one *is immune.*

This essay is about a medic who carries an ambulance call clearly in her mind, heart, and soul. Although the emotional wounds have mostly healed, the memory remains, and she is forever changed. Angel is now 33-years-old with several years' experience as a trauma center ER Tech. The medic became an ER RN who worked in the trauma center with her daughter; apple does not fall far from the tree. What a legacy.

Sweet Dreams, Angel

The telephone's ringing was an unwelcome intrusion into the night, breaking our silence into a thousand shards reflecting bits of dreams and pieces of reality mixing into an unreachable moment.

"Station nine, Cheryl,*" I mumbled, feigning coherence and attempting to ground myself at the moment and comprehend the directions I was about to be given.

"Priority one," said Ronda,* the EMS dispatcher. "I need you on the air right away."

I shook off the last remnants of sleep and called out to my partner in the bunk beside me. "Bob*: priority one. Ronda sounds a little edgy—we'd better move it."

---

* Some names have been changed. The first time such a name appears in the text, it is marked with an asterisk.

Sometimes the dispatchers have to use creative management skills when the crews on 24- hour shifts rebel at sporadic and interrupted sleep. Working a double, this had been one of those shifts. We were trying to grab a quick nap and had missed lunch and dinner.

Company policy dictated that we had three minutes to get into the ambulance and report on the air after contact with dispatch. Instead of using our time to freshen up, we each popped a piece of chewing gum into our mouths and immediately headed out the door. We assumed that Ronda was in a mood and did not want to incur further wrath. We still had 10 of the 48 hours left to work and alienating the affections of a dispatcher can never result in anything positive for EMS crewmembers.

"Alpha 255 is on the air."

"255, priority one for Dearborn Park. Make northbound Southfield ramp to I-94 westbound. Child hit by a van. Your D-card number is 3472, time of call 2209h."

"Alpha 255 copies."

We understood the edginess in Ronda's formerly calm voice. The big three in dreaded EMS calls are those involving family members, friends, and children. Normally I drove and Bob navigated, but this was a race against time. Bob jumped in the driver's seat, and I hopped into the back of the rig to set up the advanced life support equipment. We had known before we pulled the ambulance out of the bay that when a pedestrian takes on a motor vehicle, the vehicle usually wins.

"Spike two lines, normal saline and lactated ringers," yelled Bob over his shoulder, straining above the screaming sirens. I knew what to do, but Bob calling out orders and my responding as I completed each step began the process of communication that was vital to our success as a team. "Pull out the drug box and set up the (cardiac) monitor. Don't prepare the paddles or leads until we see how big this kid is."

I hung the bags, though it seemed to take an interminable time. My hands felt big and especially clumsy as I tried to pull the packaging open and bleed the IV lines. The overhead strobe lights cast eerie red intermittent bursts inside the patient compartment, ticking off the seconds in our patient's Golden Hour.

It triggered an almost comical mental image of a wino, sitting in a cheap hotel room, and chain-smoking cigarettes with eyes transfixed on a small black-and-white TV screen. In this image, a red hotel sign flashed just outside his window, giving momentary peeks into the red, smoky glow of his reality. At that particular moment, my reality was just as undesirable. I tried to free myself of those images to accomplish my tasks, taking a deep breath to reduce my anxiety and approaching panic.

"Both bags are hung, the tape is ripped and hanging on the overhead bar. Catheters are in a box on the bench seat with the pulse oximeter, and the oxygen is on. Do you want the intubation kit left in the jump kit or opened and set up back here?"

"Leave it in the jump kit," said Bob. "We might have to tube him on the ground."

It was hard for me to monitor the radio communications from the back of the rig, so I asked Bob if the fire department was on the scene: his response was a brusque, "Affirmative." We knew that if fire-rescue workers were already there, they would stabilize our patient and perform whatever basic life support measures necessary. The fire trucks were a welcome sight as we rounded the curve toward the scene of the accident. My anxiety reduced slightly as I mentally checked off items in the victim stabilization process. Firefighters on scene completing primary steps permitted us to leap into advanced trauma and life support measures that could increase our patient's chances for survival.

At that moment before stopping the rig and beginning our tasks as paramedics, I switched to a more emotional appraisal of the situation. It is not our job to judge patients or their circumstances, but maintaining that particular level of professionalism is extremely difficult when you see severe trauma to a child. You cannot help wondering what prompted the child to be in such a dangerous place, especially at night.

And where were his parents? Did they not care enough to monitor his whereabouts or bear any concern for his safety? Did they just assume that he had the appropriate judgment at his age to take care of himself?

Somehow, I switched into an empathetic mode for the child and anticipated grief and loss. In my denial, I allowed a moment of anger before I saw the boy's face or condition. Inwardly, I prayed for this to be a salvageable situation. We stopped the rig. The doors, pulled open by the firefighters, revealed a scene I had hoped not to see.

Looking at our patient, it did not seem like anyone would ever have the opportunity to question his judgment, or take away some privilege as punishment for his playing in traffic. The boy was obviously paying the price for what was probably an impulsive act. Instead of worrying about things that normally concern kids—like cool clothes, catching something awesome on the tube or getting the latest computer gadgetry—this kid was struggling to breathe.

The fire department rescue crew had already applied MAST pants to stabilize lower extremity fractures and secured our patient to a long backboard. He appeared about 10-11 years old, blonde hair, about 5 feet tall, maybe 95 pounds. There were multiple abrasions on his head and face, matting his blonde hair into bloody clumps, with bruising around both eyes. Blood oozed out of the boy's nose and mouth, staining the cervical collar placed around his neck by the firefighters. He was in labored, agonal respirations as we approached him.

Bob checked for pulses and found a faint radial pulse at a non-life-sustaining rate of about 30. The boy's pupils were fixed and dilated, his skin cool and pale, and his lungs were already filling with fluid. We popped an airway in his mouth and began bagging with 100% oxygen. Lifting him onto our stretcher, we welcomed him into our world: a guaranteed, miracle-making, emergency room on wheels, prayers administered copiously at no extra charge.

Come one, come all, see the happy ending, just like on TV. No one dies, and no one is permanently impaired. Somehow, just before the final scene, the heavens open, music sounds, and all are well.

After loading, we again checked for a heartbeat. Confirming that the boy was pulseless and not breathing, Bob muttered an expletive and called for CPR. A firefighter jumped in the front seat of the ambulance to drive. While the firefighters on board continued compressions and bag-valve-mask ventilations, we got the intubation equipment ready.

A quick-look on the cardiac monitor showed an AMF rhythm (*Adios, Mother F—r*), also known as asystole—flatline. Firefighters continued CPR with hyperventilation while Bob intubated and I looked for a site to gain IV (intravenous) access. We knew the prognosis was not good, but neither of us was good at accepting failure or seeing a situation as impossible. We had the skills and the toys. Somehow, we would make it work. We had to, as defeat and loss were not acceptable options.

The firefighters already cut the boy's thick left coat sleeve. I assumed they had prepared an opening for me to start the IV line and I grabbed the boy's arm with both hands to look for a good vein. The upper left arm bent quickly in half like a rag doll, mid-shaft. Apparently, his humerus had sustained a complete fracture, and the arm bent grotesquely and flopped off to the side.

I shuddered, took a deep breath to decrease my nausea, grabbed my medic shears, and cut away the thick coat sleeve on the other arm. Finding an acceptable vein, I muttered an audible and brief prayer, something like, "Dear God, please let me get this first try," and popped a needle into his right antecubital vein. I taped the line down as Bob secured his endotracheal tube, and started preparing the drugs while Bob established a second line in the boy's external jugular vein.

Things moved smoothly and efficiently, like a well-rehearsed movie scene. It felt like an aberration of time to me as sounds and movements achieved a slowing distortion. Our on-scene and en route times would later prove exceptionally brief, but as we performed our duties, it felt as though we were there for eons.

Every thought and movement jumbled together, feeling thick and expanded as one might view the world through the feverish eyes of illness. Despite perceptual conflicts, we managed to get weak pulses back after pushing the epinephrine and atropine, which gave us momentary hope to pull this child out of death's clutches and back into his mother's arms. As we worked against time and mortality, the monitor showed an ever-hopeful sinus tachycardia at a rate of 120, but it did not last.

During the call, we pushed all of the appropriate drugs and performed our protocols flawlessly but the boy, whose name we later learned was Scott,* died at the hospital. His skull exhibited profound crepitation and his abdomen was rigid and distended with spilled blood. My partner wrote the report as I cleaned our rig with Big Orange, a delightfully fresh aroma designed to replace the smell of blood and other spilled bodily fluids with a more socially acceptable citrus scent.

When we finished, I went back into the ER and held onto Scott's cold foot. Our training concentrates on producing positive results and saving lives. Nobody ever told us what to do when our advanced skills and expensive toys do not work.

No one ever explained that you could be completely successful in applying your talents and still come out with the worst result. No one ever walked us through how to handle it emotionally when a child dies. No one seemed to be there for the medic feeling lost, hopeless, and helpless, watching the spirit of a child fade into the universe.

Bob and I did not talk about Scott, or the call, except to review the procedures. There was nothing we could have done differently, but the boy died. I reminded myself that God performs miracles in His time and on whom He decides to confer them. Scott was not to be a recipient. My partner and I finished our shift and without another word, went home.

I spent the next several hours cuddled up with my daughter. I phoned my son and told him I loved and missed him. The ambulance call, every detail perfectly preserved—a video without end—played itself continuously in my head like a promotional loop. It was a song that keeps repeating itself in your consciousness, getting louder and louder and you cannot escape from it. My heart raced, and I could not take one of those deep, cleansing breaths that reduce stress to offer some measure of relief. There was no relief. There was no return to normalcy.

Sometimes, in a hidden corner of the mind, there exists a place removed from reality. Darkness and the images that saturate the senses reaffirm an individual's powerlessness. These images are beyond the point of chosen exposure or experience.

I spent the next 48 hours unable to eat or sleep, reliving the recent violation with its unrelenting intrusive thoughts following the trauma. As the second night filled with darkness devoid of mercy, the line between rational and irrational thought became a chasm leading to an emotional abyss. I reached out for help.

Mark D. is a good friend who holds a degree in psychology. When I called him, a friend of his answered the phone, telling me that Mark had just stepped out. "This is Cheryl. It's nothing important, really, not a matter of life and death. Well, I guess it is about life and death, but it's no big deal. Just tell Mark I said hi."

He called back within minutes.

"What's going on?"

"I had a bad call. We picked up a kid who had been FUBAR'd (F—d Up Beyond All Recognition) by a van. I don't know what the deal is because I've been doing this for years, and nothing has ever really bothered me before, but I can't eat or sleep or turn it off, and it just keeps rolling around in my head."

"All right. First of all, I have a lot of respect for what you do. I could never do it. What you do and what you see out there are not the normal things that people see, or should see. Tell me what happened."

Quickly relating the call in elaborate detail with the images so firmly imprinted in my mind and heart that I could effortlessly rattle them off without stopping to breathe, I told Mark what happened. I could not catch my breath, and the room seemed to swim as I visited that place. My senses relived their experience: the smell of exhaust and blood, the bits of glass crunching under my boots, the controlled panic in the eyes of the emergency workers as they fought so desperately against death.

Feelings of inadequacy mounted, accompanied by the urgent desire to quit my job. I did not want to face parents handing me dead babies or have to wonder, racing against time to a scene, what I might find. There was a wave of understanding beginning to flow over me.

The medics with whom I have worked told, in their most private moments, of a desire to have the power of God, just once, to re-inflate a soul with life in the middle of senseless tragedy. I had yearned for that power even if it meant just giving Scott's parents the time to hold him and say goodbye before his body grew cold and lifeless. I had far more questions than answers, but could not identify or speak them as my heart ached with this loss.

Mark listened patiently. After I had answered all of his questions, he asked the one that opened the door of my prison. "What was different about this call?"

It took a few minutes to understand what he was asking. I had seen people in pieces, handled drowning victims, offered comfort and understanding to those who faced a loss of dignity and sanity. I had been the recipient of projectile vomitus, perceived as a hero, and then scorned, all on the same day. What was different about this call was not the call itself.

I was in the middle of some demanding personal problems. That same day, my (now) ex-husband had stormed out of the house, refusing to watch our 10-year-old daughter and leaving her to fend for herself. At work and away from home I was powerless to care for her and hoped that the neighbor she was visiting, Lynn, would see to her safety.

I had assumed she was safe as she rode her bike with her friends down our quiet streets, but I could not justify that assumption. There is no safe place. There is no place where the boogeyman is forbidden, where pain, sorrow, and loss will not enter and change everything we know in ways we could never imagine.

The anger at my situation and the realization of the parallel between the family of the dead child and my own became clear. Scott's mother left him with relatives trusting that he would be safe. I was with this other mother's child as he took his last breath and died.

Where was my child during this time?

I remembered suppressing a horrible fear as I fought for Scott's life. What if another medic was cutting my daughter's coat sleeve, looking for a good vein, trying to instill life into her lifeless form? Would they mourn her loss? Or would they be callous and marvel simply at how physical trauma can pull apart a human body without giving a thought to the soul?

Would they know my daughter was a beautiful little girl who excelled in gymnastics and played trumpet? Would they suspect she decorated cakes and was a whiz at reciting Bible verses? Would they know what she would miss, what I would miss, in a future now denied her?

Mark let me see that I was crying for this dead child, and my child, for any pain in her life I could not control, for any moment lost I could not regain. I could feel Mark's hand leading me gently out of the darkness of my emotional prison. I cried for Scott and his family, prayed for their strength through each coming day, and felt a release as I let him go.

My daughter was upstairs in her bed, asleep. After hanging up the phone, I stood over my baby girl and just watched her for a while. Her breathing was deep and even, her face as sweet and innocent as a newborn. Thanking God for her, and for Mark's wisdom and kindness, I climbed into her bed and wrapped my arms around her. Tucking her warm feet between mine, and whispering, "Sweet dreams, Angel" into her ear, I drifted off to sleep.

~~~

As *EMS professionals, we do not discuss some things publicly because the outside world would not get it. They might judge us as crude, callous, insensitive, or uncaring. However, sometimes our lives overflow with blood, guts and gore, trauma and tragedy, and insane hours without food, sleep, or solace. We are "Ambulance Drivers" judged as having no more skills than the fella who asks, "Would you like fries with that?" (No offense intended to the fast-food employees who keep us alive.)*

The following story is one of those 'you had to be there' disclosures, the gallows humor used by emergency services personnel. When we stop laughing, we cry, so finding a humorous moment in any situation is the key to our survival. Besides, you just cannot make this stuff up.

Cheap Date

In a very small town bordered by Lake Michigan,* everybody knew everybody and the town folks often wore multiple hats. For example, the Police Chief, "Jr,*" was the EMS Director/Police Chief (Medical Examiner, local auctioneer, farmer, and real estate agent). Police were Emergency Medical Technicians (EMTs) of varying licensure.

The EMS service was housed within the police station. The building was small, and the EMS quarters were in a minuscule room off the front desk of the police station, consisting of a bunk bed, small refrigerator, table, and shared coffee pot. There was no distance between the officers and EMTs, physically or emotionally.

In the PD/EMS community refrigerator, you might see a container of yogurt sitting apathetically next to a sealed box containing tubes of blood, as the police chief/ME held evidence samples awaiting transport to the sheriff's office. The shared bathroom had no shower. Those who worked 48-hour shifts learned to make do with grooming and hygiene accomplished in the sink. Former strangers became family, albeit shirttail relatives, in a hurry.

Most of the EMS staffers were volunteers who responded from home via pagers dispatched from the county seat several miles away, avoiding the need to *live in* during their shifts. It was an exciting experience to work in this city teeming with lively characters and infinite stories. Whether the uniforms were police blue or EMS gray, the officers and EMTs worked as a team.

Dispatch information was often sketchy and guarded because most townsfolk owned scanners and monitored radio calls. The county dispatcher sent out police, fire, and ambulances. Most locals kept a tablet next to the radio to take notes, allowing them to pass the information along to their neighbors. If they did not know the police 10-codes by heart, they often had a cheat sheet under the scanner box for quick reference.

On one call, the primary county EMS unit, Alpha 93, dispatched to a private address for an unknown medical emergency, which could mean anything from someone falling out of bed to a full arrest requiring CPR and advanced life support. A police unit, ambulance, and several volunteer EMS personnel responded to this scene within minutes.

Alpha 93 paramedics arrived to find a 54-year-old male, whom we will call Marcus,* sitting on the toilet. Police came shortly after that and found one paramedic, Roy,* standing next to the patient and the other, a female RN/Medic named Sasha,* on her knees with gloved hands closely examining the patient from the front. When the police officer, John, viewed the nature of the medical emergency, he quickly made eye contact with Roy,* visually relaying, "I cannot believe what people do." John did his best to stifle laughter, only letting go of a polite and forced cough or two. He turned his head to let his face relax for a moment before coming back into view of the patient and the rest of the crew.

The strain of holding a straight face for an extended period was becoming painful. Officer John realized he was about to lose control and break out into the type of laughter that leaves one breathless and makes their sides ache. John excused himself and went to the front yard to redirect other EMS volunteers arriving from home.

No further assistance was needed. Everything was under control. Move along. We packaged and loaded the patient onto the EMS stretcher with care and transported to the closest appropriate hospital. Following the guarded radio report during transport, the staff received a more detailed face-to-face accounting in the ER.

Apparently, the male patient had been pleasuring himself into a sample-sized bottle of shampoo, and the bottle was stuck— for two days. Thinking that the situation would resolve itself, the man did not seek medical attention until the pain became excruciating. The man's genitals swelled to the point of almost engulfing the shampoo bottle with a purplish-red and fluid-filled hunk of flesh that was, and with luck would be again his penis.

In small towns, one incident trumps another. The crews discussed current EMS calls during weekly continuing education sessions intended to increase their knowledge base and treatment options.

Although we learned from the experience, Marcus' rendezvous with the shampoo bottle became a medical memory.

We responded to many interesting calls in that town. We went into the woods where migrant farm workers gathered for a woman who began seizing while chanting in tongues over an animal sacrifice. A man had gotten into a car accident, and when the paramedics delivered him to the ER, his mother screamed about cutting away expensive clothing to treat the patient's life-threatening wounds. A self-inflicted gunshot wound to the leg resulted from a kid cleaning the gun he purchased to protect himself, as "you never know who might come up from the city."

We put old folks back into bed, assured the woman who woke up with a dead husband, who probably died several hours before, that he must have *just* passed away because he was still warm (under the electric blanket). We laughed at EMT-Officer John, who, fatigued in the middle of the night, electronically sent a misleading cardiac rhythm to the hospital 30 miles away, requesting a death declaration. The doctors hesitated to declare the man as dead because the monitor showed a perfect sinus rhythm. After fussing with the monitor and arguing with the hospital staff that the man was indeed quite dead, John realized he forgot to mention that the man had a still-functioning pacemaker. Oops.

Meanwhile, someone else took a side mirror off one of the ambulances while backing up, so *please* be careful. Lastly, no more squirting Medic Shawn through the open bunk room window while he is asleep as he then has to respond to calls in a wet uniform, which is unprofessional. Oh... and please stop removing and hiding Shawn's light bar from his POV (privately owned vehicle). If Shawn wants to be Joe Medic, let him.

Several weeks later, the EMS crew and police officers who had responded to Marcus' all but forgotten rescue were walking down the street to the local café, Mom's Eats.* They saw Marcus coming out of the local convenience store carrying a full-sized bottle of shampoo. The police chief, Jr, recalling the incident from which Marcus had apparently healed, could not contain himself. As he looked in Marcus's direction, he remarked to the EMS crew (ever so casually but with an obvious glint in his eye), "Look... Marcus has a date!"

~~~

When the patient is a friend, family member, or even the casual acquaintance of a rescuer, the experience for an Emergency Services (ES) Worker changes exponentially. This story is about Regan, the neighbor of several EMTs in a small Midwestern town. Seeing bad things happen to children is the worst, knowing them is unthinkable. The ES folks who were involved in her life and death will never forget her.

Regan: Little Girl Lost

Regan* was 10 when I met her. She had flaming red hair, countless freckles, and a shy reserve that made you want to pull her out of her highly developed shell and introduce her to all the fun stuff in the world. A little overweight and terribly sensitive, Regan often hung around with my daughter, Elise,* who was only seven. Living three houses apart, Regan and Elise were convenient best friends.

Elise would invite Regan over to play and dig into the Susie Homemaker treats from our kitchen. I remember Regan giggling about having a choice of so many from-scratch goodies not readily available at her house. Regan came from a home with two brothers, two working parents, and a deaf grandmother. She seemed bashfully happy with a quick smile and subdued laugh, yet without many friends.

The last time I remember Regan visiting, it was because she had missed the bus and her mom was already gone for the day. "I don't know what to do," she said tearfully. I told her not to worry; I would drive her to school. If only all of life's' problems could be so easily solved.

At that time, I was mostly a stay-at-home mom preparing to become a volunteer EMT. Toward that end, I received the mandatory but goofy red, white, and blue smock to wear on ridealongs that blatantly identified me as a trainee. The PD/EMS Chief issued a pager allowing me to respond from home, as I lived two blocks from the ambulance bay.

The smock was forgivable because even without an EMT license, the pager and smock inspired the same level of respect given established medical professionals. If EMTs were having lunch at the local restaurant and had to run to a call, those EMTs would often return to the restaurant later to find their meal packaged and ready for take-out. Respect comes in many forms, and those small acknowledgments of personal value were one benefit to a sometimes thankless job.

The third rider is the unlicensed third person on board the ambulance, an extra pair of hands in part of *see one, do one, teach one* process. My uniform, boots, and trainee smock were at the ready, and I became adept at going from asleep to fully dressed and in my car within one minute. If I was in a very deep sleep, that minute usually included about 10 seconds of bouncing into doorways and walls while trying to orient myself to place and time. Later, I learned to snooze in a sleeping bag on top of the bed, so if awakened from a deep sleep, I would know that I was either on call for the volunteer service or at work for my city EMS job.

One night when the alarms went off, they were not just the tones from the radio dispatcher. The town sirens also rang out. There was a fire somewhere, and all emergency vehicles were to respond.

On this particular night, I was not on call to ride along, so when the town sirens beckoned, I pulled the pillow over my head and waited for them to stop. The tones preceded the information given a few moments later that I could not ignore. The fire was on the opposite side of my street and about three houses down. I pulled on my gear and walked rapidly—one must never run—across the street and toward the fire.

The first thing I saw was a volunteer firefighter holding an oxygen mask over the face of the male homeowner. The mask showed some misting, so I knew the man was still breathing, and since the ambulances had not yet arrived, I assumed the firefighter had this patient under control, and I walked toward the house. Unable to get any closer than the front yard, I returned to the dad, Gregg,* who was no longer breathing.

As I started compressions, I asked the volunteer firefighter where he had the oxygen setting, wanting to assure that the oxygen (O_2) was on high. The man answered that he did not know how to work the O_2 tank, and I discovered that the oxygen was not turned on, although the mask had been on the patients face for several minutes. I flipped the O_2 to a high-flow setting and continued CPR on Gregg as medics packaged him into ambulance number one. Gregg received advanced life support efforts, including intubation and bagging to force air into his lungs.

By this time, the mom and two sons were standing in the yard after descending a second-story window. Two people remained in the house: Grandma, who was deaf, and Regan. Firefighters searched the home.

They found the grandmother in the forward bedroom and put her into the second ambulance, which I drove to the hospital. Firefighters found Regan later in her grandmother's closet. She was not breathing by the time crews loaded her into the third ambulance.

When I finished cleaning the rig, always the newbie's job, Regan's mom, Sue,* found me at the ambulance entrance. "They won't tell me anything. I know Gregg is dead, but they won't tell me about Regan."

"Sue, I can only tell you about what happened in my ambulance. Your mom came in with us, and she was having some difficulty breathing because of the smoke, but she is doing better now. I do not know anything about Regan at this point. She was in another rig.

"I am sure the doctor will be out to see you as soon as he can, but right now, everyone is working very hard on your family. I am so very sorry about Gregg. I'm going back in to see if they need another pair of hands and someone will be out as soon as there is anything to tell you."

I lied. I had never consciously lied to anyone before, holding truth above justification of lying due to circumstance. This time, I decided to hide behind ignorance. I did not know what to say or how to comfort this mother, or if it was my place to deliver this life altering news. Surely, a doctor or some other medical professional would tell a mother something as agonizingly painful as the fact that her daughter was not coming home.

I quickly rationalized that I was not lying but simply not telling her the entire truth. It was a lie by omission, something I would have to deal ethically with later. I had already been in to see Regan, and she was dead. Her body was there, but the essence of her had disappeared, and all I saw was the soot-stained face of a little girl lost.

Like so many other children who face the reality of smoke and fire, and despite her elementary school drills and training, Regan hid in the closet. First, though, she attempted a very brave act for a 10-year-old girl. She went into her grandmother's room to alert her. Regan chose to put the safety of her family before her own and then panicked, losing her life.

Such an expression of true love, to put the needs of others first regardless of the potential cost, and this little angel did it without considering the consequences. Regan's face was so thickly covered with black smoke that the funeral director later remarked to the EMS crew, privately, that he had a heck of a time "covering that up with makeup" for the viewing. It is very sobering to see a dead child but to see one with whom you have developed a relationship is heart wrenching. To see one of your daughter's best friends laying there, knowing that you have to face your child to tell that her friend has died, is mind numbing.

I still cannot remember how I told Elise that Regan had died. I remember only that I let Elise sleep through that night because I knew her worldview would change the next morning. She needed that last bit of peace to bear the coming days.

At the funeral, the wall of blue and gray formed from police officers and EMS was impressive. The church was overflowing, so a side room opened where we all stood at attention during the services. We discreetly cried along with the other folks, but never broke rank, showing the town that they could count on us. More than duty, it represented the lifestyle and personal choices of those who wear uniforms.

At the funeral with two caskets—of a father and daughter—this trainee lost her rescuer-innocence when the caskets closed. I have never visited Regan's grave. I will remember the tender giggle and sparkling eyes in the warmth and safety of my kitchen when I was not wearing a uniform or trying to save someone's life. Just somebody's mom, doling out cookies, milk, and a diversion from the chaotic world in which I lived.

An EMT student at the time, I thought the incident and its immediate pain had passed as I continued studies toward becoming a licensed EMT. Coming early to class was a habit as I was eager to glean every bit of knowledge from the instructor, Jon. I often spent extra time before class with Jon garnering wisdom beyond the 12 hours per week of class time.

Like many with a *Rescuer Personality,* I wanted to be the best and make a difference, so I needed to prepare. I had viewed the *Faces of Death* movies for assurance that if I were going to get sick, it would be in private. Spilling my cookies at an accident site would have been an unforgivable and embarrassing act.

Jon had just completed an afternoon CPR class and was putting away his equipment when I arrived. He asked me to put the child Annie doll away into her case. A simple request and I eagerly complied.

Putting Annie into that case and closing the lid caused a flashback to the closing of Regan's casket. I completely broke down (in the bathroom, out of sight). To be an EMT you have to be tough, to buck up if you cannot handle it on your own, you are in the wrong business. Having no idea why I was crying, I stayed in the bathroom until the sobbing stopped.

When I came out 15 minutes later, Jon asked if I was ok, assuming it was some girl thing. I maintained silence and some measure of dignity with a quick smile and a muttered, "I'm fine." No one would know about my breakdown. The embarrassment of not being able to handle a tough call would escape notation in my class folder, important because I had held it together so well at the funeral.

I would go on to face other challenges. In this small town, the accepted method of coping with bad calls was to go to the Chief's house, play cards, talk about something nonsensical, and eat pie. It was not the emergency services workers' standard of care for psychological response to crisis, but it was all we had. Peer support came through sharing irreverent conversation and often-inappropriate laughter.

I suppose that was early crisis management, and for some, it seemed to work. For others, just burying and suppressing seems to work -- for a while. Eventually, it all comes bubbling to the surface with such tremendous force that the ES worker is blindsided by the hit.

Better ways to cope include peer support programs or talking to a mental health professional or chaplain. Some still reject help for keeping the pain to themselves. A sad way to live as the calls and memories build upon one another forming an emotional cache. When that loosely sealed strongbox of pain flings open, usually at the most inopportune time, it can be devastating.

Like so many in my field, I remember every child who died in my arms, children and babies who were severely or mortally injured, those given to me by a mother relinquishing her dead child to medical authorities after saying a final goodbye, and drowned children who came into my ambulance for unsuccessful resuscitation. I remember them all. I remember what they looked like, their cold skin after drowning, the blood on their small bodies from gunshot wounds, the faces that were once beautiful but then burned beyond recognition. I remember those who looked like they were simply sleeping because a parent rolled over on them in bed, accidentally snuffing out their young lives.

We perform humbling duties, especially when they involve children. Yes, I remember them all, but I knew Regan, so I remember her most vividly. This little girl lost, who was there one day and gone the next.

Elise read this story, and she cried. We still have to talk about it and someday we will. For now, I know Elise has to wonder what Regan would have looked like if she had escaped that small town, and how old she would be now. Would she have gone to college or have had children? We will never know because Regan is forever 10 years old, but we know she is happy. We can still hear her laughing.

Working the road with Paramedic Rob was awesome, especially on Saturdays. We called it Disco Saturday Night as Rob found a local radio station that played nothing but disco music. Rob and his wife Cheryl are now grandparents, which makes Rob, like me, a veteran on the road. We both have gray hair and remember when Advanced Cardiac Life Support (ACLS) was hard, and run reports were easy.

Experienced people partner with newbies holding fresh EMT licenses; ink still wet from the printer. Pairing two old folks together was a joy, and I miss bopping to songs of the 70s and 80s with a guy who knew all the words and had no objection to the fact that I could not carry a tune in a bucket.

Gross is in the Eye of the Beholder

Rob and I had been with the same EMS company since 1993, lovingly called *Comedy EMS*. I talked to Rob recently and asked, of all the EMS calls he has attended, which one readily came to mind? You never know how an EMT will respond to that question.

The recollection could involve anything from a terribly bloody scene to a touching moment involving a child. Perhaps EMTs remember a complaint about scraping a drunken driver off the road in the middle of a harsh Midwestern winter at 0300, only to find the person belligerently demanding that you go back to the snowbank and find his teeth. None of the above were even close to his story. Rob shared the following.

"I went on shift as a third rider in an ambulance at a private EMS company. We were called to a clinic to take a patient home. The patient weighed 550 pounds, was in the basement of the building, and the power was out in the middle of a hot, humid summer."

Extremely heavy patients were never on a ground floor. There was never a working elevator, either, requiring you to carry those patients up or down flights of stairs. Call it a form of Murphy's Law for EMS.

Another Murphyism is that patients who code will always have consumed a heavy meal, usually spicy and aromatic. They will regurgitate what is left of that partially digested meal all over your ambulance and sometimes onto your person. Therefore, gown up whenever possible.

Patients who insist they cannot walk will demand that you carry them up three flights of stairs and put them in their beds. Once tucked securely into bed, they will suddenly remember that they left something in the top drawer of their dresser. Magically healed and energized, they will leap up to retrieve that item, smiling, as you descend the stairs with your equipment, sore backs, and freshly bitten tongues.

Often patients will call you to take them and their five children to the hospital because they were in an accident three days ago. They are now sore from the accident and make it very clear they intend to sue ... everybody. They will not have insurance, and before you have a chance to ask their names and medical complaints, they will loudly let you know that if you intend to treat them any differently because they do not have insurance, they will sue you, too.

Patients who are Jonesing for the drugs you carry in your locked drug box will complain of chest pain. They insist they suffered a heart attack in the past and need morphine immediately. They will decline oxygen and nitroglycerine, the first-line medications for chest pain. They will be allergic to all non-narcotic pain medications like Toradol™, Ibuprofen, and Tylenol™, and will list allergies to several anti-psychotic and anti-depressant medications, giving you a clue to their medical history.

Rob adds to his story, "With the help of another crew, we struggled to carry this patient on an EMS stretcher up 14 steps. The poor woman could not get the safety belt around her enormous breasts, so they were loose on the stretcher and seemed to have minds of their own. As we grunted and strained, the patient started to lean forward on the stretcher, and her weight shift caused a load imbalance. I fearfully envisioned the patient falling, killing herself and the crewmember at the bottom of the stairs, which is a great comedic moment for the movies but not so funny in real life. We regained our balance and composure despite the heat, excessive weight, momentary distraction, and everyone slipping from sweating, successfully loading her into the rig without further incident."

Medics who complain about lifting heavy patients are not socially judgmental. Some folks think that because you choose a career in emergency medicine, you should also accept without a thought that you might become injured performing your duties. Patients often choose to deny responsibility for their behavior during their medical care and the medic's health and safety are not of concern to them.

After many years of doing both jobs (street medic and ER RN), I have four bulging and herniated discs with nerve impingement, spinal cord compression, arthritis in my spine, and nerve damage that runs down one arm and leg. Consequently, I have a negative attitude about people, capable of taking care of themselves, making unreasonable demands. For example, some decide that you will dress/undress them, lift them on and off a gurney, although they were walking minutes before, and pull them up in bed. "Sir/Ma'am, please put your feet flat on the bed, bend your knees and push." Some who expect you to pull them up from a lying to sitting position because they are too "weak" will when they think no one is looking, jump up and walk to a chair, or reach behind their gurney to grab a cell phone and snacks hidden in purses and book bags.

We are not talking about truly ill people. Those folks need help, and we give it with respect and care. We fight the frustration of demands for complete support made by people without limitations. We tire of those who feel entitled. As soon as some patients get into the medical system, from the flu to a sprained wrist, they refuse to do anything, like holding up an arm for a medic to apply a blood pressure cuff.

EMTs are not spa attendants or waiters. We are medical folks who are highly skilled and trained to work medical miracles in the most difficult situations. However, when perceived as servants, we can get a little testy.

Rob kept his cool, and the patient was doing the best she could, which made it harder on Rob. The accumulation of unpleasant circumstances rife with disagreeable smells and physical demands all piled together to make the transport rough on everyone concerned. Rob adds, "We thought the worst was over… we were wrong.

"In EMS, you always anticipate the unexpected, hoping for the best but always expecting the worst. With this particular call, the major problem with our patient happened after we were in the ambulance, readying for a 22-mile transport. This patient could not rest both her breasts on her lap, so she set one, weighing approximately 50 pounds, on my leg, as I sat across from her with my knees almost touching the cot.

"The breast, not realizing it was encroaching on my personal space as well as weighing heavily on my leg, sat in that position for the entire 22 miles. During the transport, the patient continually and affectionately stroked my hand, telling me how she had not talked to anyone in days, and so appreciated, this time, we spent together. Like the crew who lifted and carried her, the patient was sweating profusely."

If you have walked through the back of an ambulance, or been a patient requiring transport to a hospital, you know the space in the patient compartment is quite limited. There is a long bench seat with storage, the stretcher locks on to a bar on the floor, and a jump seat attaches to the back of the front cab next to wall cabinets at the patient's head. Cubbies and cabinets hold everything from extra equipment and supplies to jump kits, but the design is for anything but comfort or ease of movement.

I worked many full arrests in the back of an ambulance. Usually, an EMT is bagging the patient from the jump seat, the drug box lays open on the bench seat with supplies spread everywhere, and a firefighter is doing compressions. Sometimes a firefighter would hold onto me from behind to make sure I did not fall while dealing with needles and medications. More than once I got halfway to the hospital before hearing, "In case you are wondering who is holding on to you, my name is Mike."

I was grateful for those local firefighters. I was grateful that at my height and weight of 5'4" and maybe 107 pounds, I fit comfortably into the miniature interior of the patient compartment of an ambulance. My new partners were often skeptical because of my size, but eventually got used to seeing me and appreciated a girl who could lift. I could indeed raise my share of a several-hundred-pound patient, something that probably contributed to back problems later. For Rob, who stands considerably more than six feet tall and is a big cuddly bear of a guy, there was barely room for airflow between him and the patient's stretcher.

"When we finally arrived at the hospital, the patient was moved out of the ambulance, and my pant leg was soaked from the knee to the hip. I have experienced all types of bodily fluid exposure. People have shared their soiled selves through leaky adult diapers (sometimes bloody diarrhea), sprayed mucus, and cried on me.

"I have seen the innards of dead patients and tried to revive dying babies during my fifteen years in the field, but *this* call is still the grossest thing with which I have ever been involved. I don't know whether it was the sweat or the hand-holding that was worse. However, if you ask for my most unpleasant moment in all my years of EMS service, this was it."

We always attempt to maintain professionalism in Emergency Medicine, but there are truths we share among ourselves that the public may not understand. Rob, there may be some social sensitivity on this issue. In a time of extreme political correctness and sensitivity to the feelings of others, I guess we will have to agree to keep *this* story just between us.

~~~

EMS road stories abound. Unlike those that provoke tears, this telling will hopefully beget a chuckle or two in yet another example of how road medics get through impossible situations in the least harmful way to themselves and their patients. Please remember as you read that no patients were harmed or treated disrespectfully.

This incident was years ago, and besides, I am sure everyone involved has since gone to the dark side (desk jobs). Here is an example of how we spend 95% of our time. These are the hours not filled with the terror of trying to beat death, dismemberment, and deformity, or the loss of life, limb, and liberty. This story tells of a day in the life of a Paramedic, who chose to make the most of every moment no matter how ... crazy.

95% Boredom

Bob T. was the kind of paramedic everyone loved to have as a partner. Technically accomplished and full of fun and humor, Bob made each shift fly by with never a dull moment, entertaining himself as well as those around him. Bob was totally on target with his medical care and expertise when caring for patients.

Slight of build, dark hair and eyes, glasses, and in his early forties, Bob was approaching senior citizen road status. He was one of those people who knew the rules well enough to skirt them in a way that made life fun, and did not get himself into the type of trouble he could not talk his way out of somewhat gracefully.

Bob upgraded to a white shirt, which means he became part of management and had to conform to the image of a company man. The irreverent roadies, who have the least respect for the jobs the shirts and skirts (management) do, experience an attitude adjustment when they join the upper echelon. Rolling with the tides of change is another survival mechanism in this business because those who are rigid can paint themselves into unpleasant corners. Bob rounded all the corners and cut out a few new doors and windows.

No matter what color your shirt, white for management, colors for the street staff, any paramedic will tell you that many shifts are 95% boredom and 5% terror. The streets are unpredictable, especially in the city, and more so if your partner is a *shit magnet*, someone who draws the worst calls as though carrying a full moon in his back pocket. In the 5% of calls that required proficiency in medical knowledge and practice, Bob fulfilled his duties calmly and well.

It was the other 95% of the time that required a tweak or two. To add more interest to the day and night of a 24-hour shift, as one call blended monotonously into another, one could always count on humorous stories from Bob. The stories were mostly true, about past EMS runs, and how Bob handled them with his twist on and interpretation of policy and procedure.

Bob loved caring for patients challenged in some aspect of their mental health situation and medical history. He never abused or disrespected those folks, but had a sincere interest in their private worlds, especially when patients were off their medications, which made for lively interactions.

When both partners were paramedics, they took turns attending (providing medical care in the back of the ambulance). Not all units are staffed medic-medic, though, and sometimes a medic (EMT-P) was partnered with a lower-licensed EMT specialist (EMTS). In some cities, if your partner held a lower license, he was always the driver. The person with the higher license, by law, had to be the attendant. EMTs and paramedics alike were grateful to Bob for his preference in taking the lead on mental health transfers.

When transporting psych patients, most EMTs were uncomfortable attending. They often lacked training or experience with therapeutic conversation and behavioral emergencies. Psychology is not a clear science to most paramedics, as there is often no standard algorithm for treatment and transport.

Patients who cannot self-support breathing or pulses require CPR and advanced cardiac life support. Unconsciousness from low blood sugar buys one an IV and amp of IV-push dextrose. Broken bones receive splints and awesome narcotics as ordered by generous medical protocols or local doctors. Medical problems are easier because we have algorithms. EMTs and medics prefer following those clear, science-based directives.

Although it is no longer politically correct to use the term *psych patient*, the practice has not quite caught up to PC mandates. Moving away from the term *psych patient*, each institution has designation codes, which often note the numbers and letters of the legal document used to confine the patient for evaluation. However one describes them, patients with severe mental challenges are not that simple to treat and transport.

You may have a bipolar patient in a manic phase who could be irritable or exhibiting exaggerated euphoria. A psychotic patient may not share reality with those around him. A suicidal or homicidal patient may respond to a trigger (things that will set him off into a combative state) without warning. One 25-year-old autistic patient, with a mental age of two, will bite people who utter his (unknown to us) trigger word: "No."

Most medics are not trained to handle psych patients; just getting through those types of transports without incident is their greatest desire. Bob wanted to peek into their reality, just for a moment, to see what they were seeing and try to understand what it felt like to be on the other side. Unlike the patients' reality, it was easy for Bob to step back into sanity after the transport and continue the day as though nothing had happened.

Many years ago, because billing insurance companies was the major interest of many private ambulance services (they were a business after all), multiple psych patients rode in a single ambulance. Normally, the folks were not violent and usually sat calmly. You could conceivably take four patients in one transport sitting three on the bench seat, one on the cot, and the medic would sit in the jump seat. This allowed everyone to be strapped in, and the driver would walk individual patients into psychiatric care facilities one by one.

There was always the chance that the lone medic in the back of the rig might be exposed to some level of danger with multiple or combative patients. Although we did not have anything with which to defend ourselves besides a metal clipboard, we did have a universally understood signal in our particular service. If the medic in back sensed he was in danger, he would brace himself, yell, "Dog in the road," and the driver would slam on the brakes. Usually, this served to take the combative patient off guard and off his feet, regaining order and control to the medic who was attending those patients. Sometimes buying a moment saved patient and medic both from injury.

There are often themes in calls, whether influenced by the moon, stars, or time of year when one will hear medical people talking about abdominal pain day, stroke day, chest pain day, or *everybody is nuts* day. On one of those days described as nuts, not the large oily kernel found within a shell, Bob was in his glory. The day held the relatively easy calls of running patients from a psych holding facility to the nearby hospital for medical clearance, and then to the appropriate outlying facilities for treatment. Those transports meant a lot of paperwork.

The upside was that your uniform was usually safe from bodily fluid soiling, and you might just get a lunch and the occasional opportunity to relieve your bladder. You did not have to lug your drug box a mile and a half to the pharmacy of a local hospital for exchange as with a medical transport. Getting drug orders is great fun at first, but after a few years, it is a hassle to replace medications and clean the back of the rig.

One day Bob had four psychiatric patients. His partner, who was also his driver, happily volunteered to walk each patient into the various facilities from the rig. Bob stayed in the back of the ambulance throughout the multiple transports and drop-offs.

The jump seat faced the back of the ambulance and the head of the patient stretcher. On that day, the stretcher held a schizophrenic patient with suicidal and homicidal ideations. The patient was a flight risk, psychotic, and having suicidal and homicidal ideations, so he was restrained to the stretcher for his and the crew's safety.

The bench seat, directly across from the stretcher, held three somewhat cooperative patients. One patient was depressed, so essentially silently accommodating, and the other two very manic and verbose, both with delusions of grandeur. One thought he was Jesus Christ,* the other thought he was Pontius Pilate.* One could not write a better scenario, and Bob was eager to get points of view from their individual and collective histories.

> Bob: "So, Jesus: How does it feel to sit next to Pontius Pilate?"
> Jesus: "I have forgiven him."
> Pontius Pilate: "Forgiven me? I didn't do nothing wrong! And I don't need your forgiveness; I didn't put you on no cross."
> Bob: "So you've washed your hands of the whole thing, eh Pilate?"
> Pontius Pilate: "I asked if he was the King of the Jews and he answered blasphemy. I didn't cut him; I didn't spill his blood!"
> Jesus: "You don't know the truth."
> Bob: "So, Pontius can't handle the truth! Pontius, have you ever met Jack Nicholson?"

The conversation continued until Pontius Pilate, Jesus, and the silent person (possibly Judas Iscariot) arrived at their respective facilities. The patient on the stretcher was last. His delivery required that both medics leave the ambulance and escort the patient into the facility together.

The psychotic patient had told the medical doctors that he was hearing voices commanding him to harm himself and others. Since the patient had been off his medications for several months, the doctors could not assure the patient's safety in anything but a lock down facility. Every few minutes during the transport, Bob would watch the patient turn his head to the side of the ambulance holding the supply cabinets, nod, mumble a few words that Bob could not understand, and then return to a non-blinking forward stare.

Bob and his driver gained entrance into the locked building to deliver their final patient. They moved him by stretcher into the elevator, noticing something that had, for them and their multiple trips to that facility, blurred into the background noise. The elevator verbally announced the direction of the elevator, the floors it crossed, and upon which floor it finally stopped -- in a female voice. The patient tensed at the voice each time the elevator spoke, aware that the EMTs beside him were both males.

As Bob and his partner off-loaded from the elevator, the patient nervously looked around to locate the female whose voice he heard. Whether the patient understood what the voice had relayed was unknown to the partners. The moment the patient peeked back into this world, a lone female voice caused his discomfort. When the patient looked to Bob for an explanation, the patient saw a half-smile as Bob, whistling, pulled the stretcher forward without comment.

Peeking into the additional confusion caused by a disembodied voice hovering over his patient, Bob sighed in relief at the simplicity of his world. Bob stepped back into the comfort of his knowing, a more authentic existence, where he treasured the contentment of two feet on firm psychological ground. At the end of the shift, home, family, and a common experience of shared reality awaited him.

~~~

My name is Sherry, and I am a Trauma Junkie. Because of the association with ER, EMS, and CAP, I place myself in emotional harm's way almost every day. Keep dipping your toe in the water and eventually, your whole body gets wet. I almost drowned.

Anticipation can be a greater stressor than the actual event. Although initially stress provoking, sometimes the event turns out to be a piece of cake. The ES worker walks away with the perception that this was a really cool thing to happen, a really cool place at that particular time, and it had a really cool outcome. Maybe that is the key. When it all goes well and has a positive or successful outcome, we get to be a hero, even if only for a moment, and we remember why we got into this crazy business.

Trauma Junkie in the Air

When I moved to Las Vegas, the trauma junkie in me still commuted every couple of months to continue working in a Detroit trauma center. It is in my blood, my lifestyle, a part of who I am, to continue in Emergency Medicine. I became too old and injured for the physical demands of the road, so like many medics, I moved inside.

Though I still loved EMS the most, I had to settle into the questionably comfortable lunacy of an ER. Accumulating 10 years' experience there, it felt like home. Then I moved 2,000 miles west. The decreased excitement of a more stable environment in Nevada required extensive emotional adjustment.

I was having withdrawal symptoms. Old shows provoked nostalgia, like TLC's, *Trauma: Life in the ER,* which at one point featured the places and people with whom I had worked in Detroit. Missing the action worsened when I got a quick email from Dr. Don Benson or Dr. Marson Ma, two fellows who taught me more than I ever learned from books.

During one of those trips back to Detroit, I was nestled into my coach seat, on the aisle, laughing along with two female passengers in my row who seemed as crazy as I am. It is not often that airline-assigned traveling companions are those with whom you would care to have anything but the briefest verbal exchanges. This plane's departure was delayed, annoying when you are facing a 4-hour flight. So, as we sat in the stationary plane, we passed the time in polite conversation.

We talked about different airports around the country. We detailed the types of people you meet or end up sitting beside, during your flights. We laughed about how a group of passengers *leaving* Las Vegas is often not as sophisticated, or clean smelling, like those on flights going *into* Las Vegas. The combination of smoke, alcohol, and body odor of persons coming off a multi-day gambling binge can make their seatmates long for nose plugs.

On those flights you also run into, or overhear, the folks who did the hair, makeup, nails, shopping for (or partied with) someone famous, which invokes upon them (they think) instant celebrity. They must loudly assert that association to anyone within earshot, perhaps to elevate themselves above the common society from which they have risen. McCarran International Airport (LAS) in Las Vegas is fraught with those and other characters. One might not elect to spend time with them if given a choice. Most are simply innocuous visitors coming in to have a good time and fulfill the commercial destiny of *what happens in Vegas stays in Vegas.*

It is true, especially on red-eye flights leaving Vegas, that you might risk sitting next to someone who enjoyed the active day-into-night life for several days straight without the benefit of showering. We three girls chattered about crying babies; young people who like to kick the seat behind you; and parents who let their children roam the aisles or throw tantrums. We discussed people who loudly and endlessly share details of their vacation/wedding plans/career move/next big sale with strangers who don't need, want, or know what to do with that information. On a trip back from Cancun recently, I sat across the aisle from a LOUD woman who, as a therapist, took an interest in every detail of her seat member's personal life. She loudly delved into his childhood and marriage woes. As we shared air travel stories, an announcement came overhead.

"If there are any medical personnel on board, please signal for a flight attendant."

Conversations stopped as everyone wondered, some aloud, what the medical emergency might be or who might respond. I held my breath for a moment, keeping to myself the standard utterance in those types of situations: "Oh, shit." I waited for an eternity of about 15 seconds hoping that someone else would ring his or her bell.

Responding to a medical emergency in flight is the most unpredictable of circumstances. You have no idea what the situation is, what the protocol might be, especially if you have never responded to an air emergency. You do not know about the liability in providing medical care without a physician present, what supplies they have on board, who provides the medical control authority, and how in blue blazes would you get in contact with them? No one else signaled.

I rang the bell.

When the flight attendant, Annie,* came to my seat, I said that I was a Trauma Nurse/Paramedic and asked how I might help. Annie smiled gratefully, asked me to follow her, but told me nothing until we were standing in front of a woman who was seated forward of first-class just behind the doors to the flight deck. The middle-aged female patient was pale, diaphoretic, breathing rapidly, moaning, and clenching her upper stomach. She was in obvious pain and distress. The patient, Mrs. Hua,* told me she was having extreme abdominal pain and chest pain that radiated to her left shoulder, was dizzy, nauseated, she had thrown up once already, and was having difficulty breathing.

We gave Mrs. Hua oxygen while I obtained a stethoscope and listened to her lungs; she was moving air. At my direction, Annie laid blankets on the floor for Mrs. Hua to lay down in the small space normally used as an area for first-class food preparation. Lay down before you fall down is always a good rule of thumb.

As I continued with my physical assessment and obtained a medical history, I put Mrs. Hua on a cardiac monitor and obtained vital signs. Her cardiac rhythm showed abnormalities and her physical presentation was concerning and warranted medical intervention. I asked Annie to get me in touch with medical control to obtain orders from a physician.

First, Annie followed my requests to make Mrs. Hua comfortable on the floor and prepared her for medical intervention. Then Annie located the plane's medical kit while I went to the flight deck and used the pilot's headgear to contact a physician at the Mayo Clinic. The rules have changed since September 11, 2001. New protocols prevent anyone outside of the flight deck from using the radio for the sake of higher security. This requirement complicated our attempts to handle the medical end of our emergency expeditiously.

The pilot, Captain Murakami,* knowing he had a medical crisis that required diverting his plane to the closest airport, was in touch with ground control. Sharing the microphone and radio with the captain, I tried to give a report to the Mayo Clinic and understand, as well as repeat, the orders given to me. Captain Murakami and I handed the headset back and forth as radio traffic stepped on each of our transmissions. Finally, after multiple attempts and partial communications, we each understood our orders and proceeded with them.

I returned to my patient and began pulling supplies out of the airplane's emergency medical kit in preparation for completing my orders. I asked Annie to record what I told her since the times of med-ication administration, and vital signs before and after the medications could be useful information to the crew that would assume care of the patient. Any medic who has ever trashed the back of an ambulance while trying to save someone's life (making a mess is the least of your worries) will appreciate my discarding items as quickly as I used them into a large pile. Annie attempted to control the growing mess while performing her recording duties.

The first-class cabin collectively gasped when I pulled the cap off the IV catheter, holding the needle up to the light to check for imperfections before bending down to insert it into the patient's vein. I stifled a giggle as I glanced toward them and realized I had the full attention of a captive audience. I established the IV (intravenous line) despite the turbulence and close, inadequately lit quarters. As any frequent flyer will tell you, turbulence in a sea of air, like waves, can be quite choppy.

As I taped down the IV, another flight attendant told me there were two women on the plane who identified themselves as nurses and were offering their services. The offer came a little late, but I asked the flight attendant to find out what kind of nurses they were. I did not want to overcrowd the limited space with folks who would only be in the way. I knew that if they were not well versed in emergency medicine, they probably would not be terribly helpful.

The flight attendant returned telling me that the nurses said they "knew ACLS" meaning they had taken a class and passed the certifica-tion for Advanced Cardiac Life Support. They were probably not going to be of much help unless I needed extra hands for CPR, which was hopefully not going to happen. I thanked the flight attendant and told her that everything was under control, but if the patient coded (went into cardiopulmonary arrest), I would appreciate their assistance.

I pulled out the medications and gave them to the patient as ordered. Her vital signs stabilized, and her heart rhythm returned to normal. I hung her IV fluid on a hanger (sorry first-class, one coat probably had to double up with another), then returned to the flight deck for a final communication with the Mayo Clinic using Captain Murakami's radio.

One final medication was ordered and given, and the patient and I settled on the floor as we awaited landing in Nebraska, somewhat out of the way for a flight from Las Vegas to Detroit. The patient was in a much-improved condition and began to question whether a diversion to Nebraska was completely necessary. Annie laughed and said to the patient, "Of course you feel better. You just got a ton of medicine; I'm not so sure you would be doing that well without it."

I echoed her sentiment, knowing diagnostics and possibly further treatment would be necessary. Besides that rationale given to the patient, the fact remained that in the world of medicine, one cannot initiate emergency medical intervention and then just let the patient go without turning them over to a higher level of care. It is unwise, irresponsible and possibly malpractice.

As we waited for landing, I listened to some of the conversations around me. Folks who had been complaining about waiting for a delayed takeoff, the lack of pillows, blankets, and the reduction of types of snacks provided in years past suddenly had no complaints. I cannot help but think that they were wondering what kind of care they might have gotten in similar circumstances if they had become acutely ill, had a heart attack, or cardiac arrest, or if someone they loved had taken ill on an airplane.

No one anticipates that anything will go wrong when in generally good health. An airplane ride is simply transportation between points A and B. When folks are in the air, there is no ER a convenient 5 minutes away, and medications and staffing are quite limited.

The airlines do not guarantee medically trained personnel on flights. Additionally, the flight attendants do not have training in advanced levels of medical care, and their drug boxes are limited and somewhat primitive. The entire airplane came together in support of our efforts to assist a woman who had started her day out like any other, never anticipating that something would go terribly wrong.

As we prepared for landing the flight attendant who had expertly assisted during the rescue, my new friend Annie, asked if I wanted to buckle up in one of the jump seats during the landing. I opted to stay with my patient. I knew I could hold Mrs. Hua steady, protect her IV line, and keep her from further harm if I was with her. I held on to her while bracing my back and legs against the walls on each side of her.

It was a rough landing, but we made it without incident or injury. The EMS crew was waiting at the gate. As soon as the doors opened, one medic took my report while the other two loaded the patient onto their stretcher for transport to the closest hospital.

Having worked on an ambulance for almost 10 years, I knew what the medic wanted to know and in what order. The report given to him was rapid and succinct. I also gave him the paper that documented medication times, the patient's responses, and her vital signs along the way.

Annie later said that the paramedic told her Mrs. Hua had been in the best possible hands. The medic and Annie discussed how they had only one other person "so qualified" on an in-flight rescue "in many years." The medic had asked Annie about my credentials.

"Is she a doctor? Because she knows what she is doing." That rare but dearly appreciated pat on the back adds tremendously to the success of the medical interventions. We all have egos, though rarely stroked in a world where we only hear complaints.

I gave the flight attendant two business cards naming Lt. Col. Sherry Jones, CAP, because they held my current contact information. I carried one card each for the Michigan and Nevada addresses and phones. The cards noted RN license numbers for both states, Michigan medic license number, and current applicable certifications.

For the remainder of the flight, the folks on the plane probably mentally reviewed a myriad list of difficulties they would face when landing in Detroit. Many would miss connecting flights, rides home, and appointments. The two hours of delay in Nebraska, taken up by the paperwork surrounding the rescue, restocking of supplies, and refueling, were met with silence and full support. Upon completion of documenting and signing forms for the airline (what did we ever do without paper trails?), I returned to my seat and tried to melt into the blur of passengers.

In very few minutes we were back in the air, and movement in the cabin resumed. Annie came back to my seat and generously offered two bottles of wine as a gift of gratitude from the first-class passengers. Many of them had a front row seat for all that had occurred, and Annie added their apologies for not standing and singing, "Hail to the Chief." I did not understand the reference to the military anthem until I looked down and realized I was wearing one of my favorite travel shirts, this one from Luke Air Force Base.

The rest of the flight went without incident, and as we landed, Annie added a bit of information not often heard in a landing announcement. "Our special thanks to Lt. Col. Sherry Jones, who did a tremendous job with our sick passenger." The entire plane erupted into applause, shouting, "Free tickets! Free tickets!" Annie got back on the microphone in response, stating, "Gee, and all she asked for was an upgrade!"

Again, laughter put people who might have been very tense relaxed, at ease, and added to their sense of bonding. All of the passengers calmly and politely deplaned. Everyone left feeling good about what had happened during their flight.

As I looked back on that flight, I realized that it had the potential to go in any direction, but something that could have been emotionally traumatizing for many people ended up being quite powerfully positive and motivating. I had more fun that day than I remembered having in a very long time. There is something exhilarating about doing (at that time and in that place) what nobody else there could do. If any of my EMS/ER coworkers had been present, I am sure they would have done the same thing. It just happened to be my turn.

I did not get a free flight out of the air carrier, though that might have been a nice reward. This is just what we in Emergency Medicine do, what we enjoy doing. Having everything turn out well is its own reward.

Folks watch this stuff on TV all the time, but I wish you could walk in our shoes for just a day. I wish you could know how rewarding it is to stand and face an unseen adversary, then beat him. It does not get much better than that.

~~~

It is hard to imagine what one might do when faced with someone else's death. We see death all the time on TV and the Internet, but I do not think anyone has a clue how they will react in person. How would you respond to the sounds, sights, smells and touch of the lifeless form of a body that was, only hours before, alive? How would you handle being witness to the end of someone who had their entire lives ahead of them, someone who had plans and hopes and dreams?

What would you think as you went through the motions of trying to save a life you know from the depth of your soul was already gone? How would you depersonalize it enough to do your job as a rescuer, especially if this was your first code? I thought that after all the months of EMT training, I would click into autopilot and remember the necessary steps without hesitation, that we would save the life and share good news with the family later. It does not always happen that way. To be honest, it rarely happens that way, and a save is the exception, not the rule.

Jeff Washington

I will never forget his name. I cannot remember the names of recent coworkers without great concentration and effort, but even though this call happened almost twenty years ago, I can still remember *his* name. Jeff Washington.* His face is a blur, but parts of him—his cold skin from being immersed so long at the bottom of the cold river and the way his hair matted on his head—are still as clear today as the day he died.

The Memorial Day parade had just finished. The entire local EMS crew, which was the largest and most advanced in the county, had participated. It was a very small town, so each of the three ambulances, staffed by two or three crew members, proudly participated in the four-block procession.

The parade went down Main Street and ended in front of City Hall, the home of our ambulance bay, police station, and EMS quarters. The largest businesses in town sent trucks down the parade route carrying kids who threw candies to the parade watchers on the sidelines. Special folks in costumes walked down the center of the street's parade route, eliciting laughter from the smaller children and support from the adults who likely worked for one of the companies, or knew who was under the funny suits.

There were trucks from the sugar beet factory, the pickle factory, and the cement factory, the biggest hometown employers. Visitors from out of town quickly discovered that if you showed up 10 minutes late to the parade, you missed it. The physical length of the parade was not that impressive even with all the emergency vehicles, fire trucks, and police cars. Each of us, fully dressed in our most nicely pressed uniforms, blew our horns and flashed our lights while waving at the same people we saw every day in the local stores and restaurants.

However, this was a holiday, a special day of celebration and recognition, so we did it up as best a small town could. After exiting the parade route, we drove our rigs into the ambulance bay, locked them up, and exchanged a few words about having completed another public service day. Then each of us headed home. Living closest to the city hall, I began the short walk toward home down a side street, passing entrances to the city park, and a bridge swinging lazily above the river that circled two sides of my small block.

The swinging bridge was a world-famous celebrity. Wedding parties and prom goers from distant places stood on the bridge, memorialized by friends, families, and professional photographers. Living just north of the bridge, we laughed about our inability to walk around the block as there were only two streets on land. Four of the houses on those two blocks, including mine, were over 100 years old. I loved the town's history.

The town was a beautiful jewel that I was fortunate to discover in my adulthood, having grown up in a very impersonal suburb of a major city. By purchasing and loving that old Victorian home with all its charms, and raising a family in the town, I had become a part of the history as well, and immersed myself in all that the home and town had to offer. The untouched pieces of nature were inspiring. I wanted to get a small canoe to let down into the river to explore this lengthy tributary beyond the known area of the bridge, which through many twists and turns flowed into another river, and ultimately into one of the Great Lakes.

The greenery and solace of that waterway were soul stirring. The peace of nature fed one's spirit with life and beauty. I imagined the river's history to be rich and full of charming stories of families and farmland and overcoming obstacles and hardships in earlier, simpler times.

However, after this holiday, in honor of those who had died in service to their country, the river changed. It senselessly took a life. How easily a romanticized version of life falls away when reality reveals hardships and lessons one is unable to avoid or understand.

The river lost most of its charm and allure that day. I never again desired to set into it or to feel its chilly, dirty water on my skin.

As I walked by the entry to the bridge over the river, I heard a woman screaming for help. Still in uniform, I diverted from my path and walked the 50 feet towards her. As an EMS Newbie, I was not sure what I might be facing. Those were the days before cell phones and 911 operators, so responding alone was an uncomfortable *what do I do now* proposition.

The woman pointed to the river. She said a boy jumped off the bridge and never came up. "Where did he jump in?" I tried to create a mental image of the spot, wrote down the number to the county dispatcher, and told her to go to the public telephone 100 feet away to call the police.

The woman ran toward the phone, and I went to the place over the bridge where she had pointed. I hoped beyond hope that the boy would surface and mentally prepared myself for performing CPR alone until additional help arrived. The river swelled that year from a lot of rain, and I heard later that kids often jumped off the bridge into the deep waters below when circumstances were optimal.

After this week of unseasonably warm weather, a few kids had made several successful jumps. On this last jump, one of the boys did not surface. The boys did not know that there had been dumping in that old river, and the bottom held everything from old lawn mowers to building materials. Speculators thought that perhaps Jeff hit one of those items, rendering him unconscious, or perhaps he had gotten himself caught up in the debris which prevented him from resurfacing.

It seemed an eternity until the police car swung by to where I was standing, and there was still no sign of Jeff. I told the officer, my friend, and coworker Paul,* what the woman had told me. I pointed to the place where she said the boy went down. Then I made a fatal error. I left the spot and took my eyes away from the point I had been watching.

I did not know that when you see someone go down in the water, you must never take your eyes off that location and should not leave it, as that is where the dive team will want to focus their efforts. We knew the county dive team would come, but did not know how to assist the divers from land. When the divers held a class on water rescue after this incident, we learned that bodies drop like a rock. The stream would not carry them away. It would leave them where last seen, at the bottom of the river.

Paul radioed information to central dispatch to get the dive team activated and alert the other police cars in the area. Mistakenly thinking that Jeff may have been knocked unconscious and then swept down the powerful pull of the bloated river, many of us traveled on foot and in vehicles along the river to the edge of town. We hoped Jeff might surface somewhere downstream. It was a warm and humid day, with the sun beating down and the humidity rising as the day wore on.

I was grateful for the lenient EMS dress code because I could wear black tennis shoes instead of boots with my uniform. Hang safety. Some of the medics who had been there forever preferred the comfort of shoes, so footwear was a personal choice item.

Anything in black was acceptable. I looked down at my shoes and wondered if they were going to melt into the pavement, grateful that they were as comfortable as they were. They were brand new, and it was my first day wearing them.

Paul and I and several other EMS/PD met with the dive team at the edge of the park near the bridge. They asked where the boy went down, and I swallowed hard trying to remember exactly where the woman had pointed. Paul had a different recollection than I did, so the dive team suited up, put a boat out on the river, and set out to find a body.

They began their search immediately below the bridge. Inwardly, they hoped they would not find the boy. Perhaps Jeff was playing a trick on his friends by ducking out under the bridge and waiting until they left before walking up the embankment and going home. Maybe he was enjoying a good laugh about having pulled off a joke on his friends. The boat sat in the middle of the river, communicating with divers in the shallow waters.

The worst thing that can happen to divers in the dark, murky waters of any body of water during a search is that they will find what they are looking for. The most difficult search is for a child. Perhaps an 18-year-old is no longer a child, but 18 is too young to die.

The diver, who found Jeff almost exactly where the woman had first pointed out to me that he had gone under and not resurfaced, says there is an almost sickening moment when you find a body. It is a sightless environment at the bottom of a dirty river, and the divers go in a preplanned grid to cover every inch of the area. They feel along the bottom and touch everything that is there trying to identify what might be human or disqualify it as not human.

In this search, they came across discarded car batteries, tires, shopping carts, blocks of cement, and pop bottles. Literally tons of debris tossed thoughtlessly into the river by people who saw their garbage contributions as anything but littering. Sometimes it was just fun to hear the *plop* as debris hit the water, so kids would stand on the bridge and find more things to toss in that black river. Some irresponsible adults covertly used the river as a convenient dumping ground.

The diver who found Jeff admits to almost recoiling with surprise and disbelief when he first felt something. Then he experienced acute nausea when he found something that felt like an arm. The diver realized he had found the boy.

An ambulance stood by in the park at the edge of the overfilled river. The divers struggled with the weight of the young man in the water, even though fueled by adrenaline and hope. They dragged Jeff from the center of that black, cold, unforgiving body of water to the assembly of ES workers gathered at the water's edge to perform the miracle of resuscitation.

Voices raised as the collection of divers, police, and EMTs each shouted to one another. They tried to determine the best way to get Jeff from his position half in the boat, to out of the water and onto the shore to the awaiting rescuers. As several of us stepped into the water at the edge of the bank and prepared to lift Jeff to dryer land, his body flopped clumsily.

His extremities danced, and his body bent everywhere a body is bendable. As we put him on our cot, I felt his cold skin through my gloves and saw how pasty it looked. Te recognition that this was a human being had to leave me before it became overpowering. I looked down just for a moment to find something emotionally safe to look at, something away from those open eyes.

The eyes looked, as one nurse described them, like fish eyes when there is no more life or hope of life in a human being. Jeff had a vacant stare, unlike anything I had seen portrayed in movies. It was more like that unexpected moment in a horror film when some young innocent opens a closet door only to find a dead body, eyes opened wide, falling unceremoniously toward her.

I looked at my shoes and thought, safely, "What a shame. Brand-new shoes and I will never be able to wear them again. They are full of water and mud, and you just cannot wash that out. Besides, tennis shoes never dry well. They lose their shape; they never fit quite the same way, and the cushioning is shot." It was enough of a diversion to allow a deep breath before I had to look up again and help hold Jeff's hands together so we could strap him onto the cot and head for the ambulance.

We started CPR right away and of course, Jeff threw up all over himself, the cot, and those nearest to him. We were steering the cot towards the ambulance's back doors when I remember jerking my hands away for a moment as Jeff threw up, trying to avoid vomit. I am not sure it was the appropriate thing to do, but it was a reaction for an untrained EMT who had never before done CPR on a person. You never know what you are going to do in extreme situations until something happens, and the instinct to avoid allowing someone to vomit on you is strong.

Sometimes even experienced medical folks are not so swift in moving away and receive all types of bodily fluids onto their uniforms. It is truly an unpleasant part of the job, but completely unavoidable. I took another deep breath, grabbed part of the cot and moved forward. The ground was initially grassy and muddy, transitioning into loose gravel and uneven terrain. The cot became increasingly difficult to handle while performing CPR, keeping Jeff on the stretcher, and moving forward at the same time.

We successfully loaded Jeff into the ambulance and did all the things our protocols dictated. Jeff was intubated; CPR continued; an IV line established, and ACLS (Advanced Cardiac Life Support) algorithms and protocols followed. We continued CPR, pushed medications, stopped, and felt for a heartbeat. It never came back.

We worked the code until we got to the hospital because lifesaving efforts do not terminate in the back of an ambulance. It is an ego thing among EMS folks. You will hear them say, "Nobody dies in my ambulance." I have said it myself many times, and it was always true. The patients were turned over to the hospital staff, and it was the doctor's responsibility to call the code, to declare the person dead in the ER.

To have someone die in your ambulance is to defy the unwritten rule that people are not supposed to die. We are to be able to help patients, and if we cannot, then we have failed. We are not good at handling failure. We do what no one else can do or would want to do because we have a self-image, very often, of being the type of person (superhero?) who is here to make a difference, to save lives, and perform miracles.

We are the front line and have the chance to provide the most hope and the most help. We have a hard time with the bad calls when things go wrong. It is not in our mindset or in our training to handle those times.

That is unrealistic, of course. The younger the EMS worker, in age or experience, the more likely he or she will have that perception of failure is not an option. The younger EMTs are often more ideological, and the newbie can set himself up for emotional failure and distress.

I was admittedly quite ideological myself when I worked that call on the day Jeff died. It was so many years ago and in a time when ES workers had to either be tough or get out of the business. The old relics (experienced EMTs/Firemen/Police) always said, "If you can't handle the stress, get a desk job somewhere."

Nevertheless, I did not know what to expect. Unmet expectations increase anxiety and my desire for a successful conclusion for all situations was a gargantuan setup for disappointment. Now I know that most cases of CPR and death are just another part of life, just another part of the workday. Most of the time.

Sometimes, for ES and ER workers, and for often unknown reasons, a call has the potential to get to us in a way we did not anticipate. The situation, the person, or maybe just the clothes they are wearing, can infiltrate our defenses. It can remind us of someone or something else, poking holes through our trauma armor. Those intrusions can reach down and touch the depths of our souls.

Why would Jeff's death leave an imprint on my heart?

I never knew anything about him. Was he a good kid, a good student, a good friend, a good son? Not that those things matter, but even though I had never heard of him before and had not thought much about him since, I remember his name.

He was my first.

~~~

2 | The Other Side of the Gurney
The Mortal Side of
Emergency Service Personnel

"When did you first want to be a paramedic/nurse/firefighter/police officer and why?" *We can probably all trace back to a single moment in time, an "Aha!" moment that sealed our fate. In my case, I knew I wanted to heal people, psychologically or physically, since I was four or five. The internal debate about the application of that desire continues.*

I knew that I wanted to be a paramedic when I saw Roy and Johnny on Emergency (1972 - 79). I was a junior in High School. That show was an epiphany for me, a leap of understanding that remained a secret until given the opportunity to pursue that career path.

Being a medic is my greatest accomplishment and the hardest job I have ever loved. Although I work primarily in nursing, I am and always will be a medic. Out of respect for active paramedics, I retired my license in 2012. This is where my personal story began.

And Puppy Dogs' Tails

Picture, if you will, a brunette pixie of a child who spent her first few years happily riding piggyback, viewing God's Creation over Mama's shoulder. Extremely shy and the youngest of four children, I received access to the greatest of secrets. There was an indisputable, undeniable truth in the magic of Merlin and Oz.

No wound was too great to heal. If things were not as we wished, something far better was yet to come. There would always be happy endings. And love conquered all.

Our biological father moved out in the summer of 1960, so we practiced do the best you can with what you've got. I did not know that we were materially deprived or different from other families because those things did not matter. What mattered to me, at four years of age, was entering any unknown without my siblings: a frightening prospect.

School was an unknown, the beginning of reality as other people knew it, unlike my own innately and creatively balanced world. Kindergarten? Get a rug and take a nap. Learn the rules and you will do fine. Two cents for white milk, three cents for chocolate.

Learning that there was an accepted algorithm for functions and behavior gave others comfort. Those restrictions frustrated the free and artistic spirit inside *me* that wanted to explore the infinite beauty and wonder of the world. That September dragged on while teachers hovered to assure the completion of tasks, focusing on behavioral order, painfully oblivious to fun or adventure. I made the best of it.

October and my fifth birthday came together. As each new day welcomed additional instruments in the forming symphony of color, my trek home changed. The pathway filled with fallen leaves and discoveries of every sort, a certain one quite unexpected.

A small dog was lying in the leaves. I reasoned that if Mom made all of my sicknesses and pain go away, then, of course, she could do the same for this poor mongrel. Any medication delivered by the hands that pushed unruly wisps of hair gently from my eyes, mended each wound, and made every hurt disappear could certainly help that puppy. I carried him home and put him in my mother's bed, carefully covering him with her clean, crisp white linens, and searched for aspirin.

Maybe I was experiencing some early stirrings of the healer within. Perhaps the innocent soul that believed in supernatural powers, who listened for sleigh bells on Christmas Eve, saw beyond the stiffened, decaying corpse that filled my arms. I do not remember what Mom said when I offered her that eyeless, mange-ridden body.

She probably disposed of it with as little outward repulsion or comment as possible. Of immediate concern to her was the child, me, intellectually ahead of her years but emotionally fragile. A child who would realize for the first time that her Mama was not omniscient or omnipotent, that a harsher reality existed than her knowledge or kisses and hugs could make *all better*.

I have since learned of a mercifully protective emotional barrier, one that holds reality at bay when we cannot command viability into a lifeless form. Despite intentions, equipment, knowledge, or skill, a child who stays beneath the cold, murky waters of Lake Huron for three hours may not live. If a van collides with an unsuspecting pedestrian, introducing catheters, fluids, and drugs into the person's veins, intubating his trachea, forcing oxygen into his lungs, and manually compressing his heart may not prolong his life.

Sometimes, however swiftly and expertly we perform functions, they may not result in what we perceive to be a positive outcome. Sometimes we cannot make things all better, a daunting realization that sets one upon other paths of introspection and growth. It also provides for personal empathy to deal with others' pain in the aftermath of trauma and loss.

That autumn afternoon was so many years ago, but in spite of the failure to obtain a consistently successful medical outcome, I am still trying to effect healing. The tools are shinier. The methods are more technologically advanced. We accept some results as being beyond mortal control.

Experience can be the harshest of teachers. Hard-learned lessons are often unforgiving, depleting an inner store of innocence. My inner child has outwardly grown and gone, and there is wonder now—and hopefully not fear—in the unknown.

I face challenges with an understanding that my younger years lacked. Somewhere I gained a forbearing. It keeps me safe and points me toward help when situations are beyond my control, understanding, or ability to handle physically or emotionally.

Maybe people desire to become rescuers because they have common personalities. The theory, though yet unproven, makes a lot of sense. I see common personality traits in the people with whom I have worked in Emergency Services (ES), whether in disaster relief, EMS pre-hospital or in the ER. Who are these people? Look around you, or look at yourself and tell me if some of this does not strike a chord of logic.

The rescuer personality is a stereotypical characterization of the types of people who work in ES. These folks often have a need to be in control of situations. Maybe they are perfectionists, lightheartedly referred to as anal or obsessive compulsive, by their families and coworkers. Perhaps they are high achievers first in school and then in life in general, internally motivated, and possibly somewhat action oriented.

They are most likely family-oriented, often considering certain coworkers close as family members, whether family by birth or choice. Whenever anything goes wrong, or someone is in need, these rescuers have an urgent desire to help, and a very hard time saying no. The rescuer personality individuals might be those who are easily bored and apt to take risks as they run toward the fire, disaster, or the bad guys instead of away from them.

You may find they have unusually high expectations, especially of themselves. They are likely very dedicated and protective with a strong compulsion to be needed. Even with these qualities, these same people will probably be so busy taking care of everyone else that they essentially come in last for self-care. There is usually not a lot of discussion about *their* needs or feelings.

Is having the dubious and controversial rescuer personality a bad thing? Not necessarily. However, it can become an obstacle when that rescuer is in need of rescuing. In the aftermath of the unsuccessful events, when his innocence is gone, and he cannot compel the desired outcome, some attributes of the rescuer personality do not leave the rescuer much room to breathe. He can become overwhelmed.

So who rescues the rescuer? Many have developed effective survival mechanisms that are usually healthy and productive. In essence, the rescuer may be in a position to apply some level of self-help, to rescue himself.

He may have enough knowledge to identify a crisis and seek outside help. In looking at the descriptions of a rescuer personality, I see myself. I see that four-year-old child who stepped through the majesty of an autumn day to face a hopeless situation that would not reverse, in spite of unassailable beliefs and expectations.

I can still see the fallen leaves and smell the crisp autumn air. I stepped into my future while lifting my first encounter with death toward a light that would eventually lead me down a different path. That light, or enlightenment, would direct my spirit to embrace thinking that let me see the wonderment on the other side of the rainbow.

Do each of us in this business have a story? Do we all experience an *Aha* moment? Is there a right-lobar burst of brain waves and information processing that gives us creative insight as to how we might spend the rest of our lives helping others? Does the business influence our personality, or does our personality lead us to the business?

Like many who choose the rescuer or healer path in life, there was also a time when I passed from inexhaustible hope to the realization that things might not always turn out right. Not everything might have a happy ending after all. During this time of reconstruction, I scribbled a note to myself, which I still have, as I tried to understand what was happening.

"There's been an invasion of sorts into my being, permeating every cell and causing a complete transformation. Since efforts to rid myself of this virus have proven futile, I wonder where this internal evolution will lead." It is a treacherous walk, sometimes, when you deal with life and death. We who have chosen that existence often have unique ways of coping with the stressors to which we expose ourselves.

I have a poster to the left of my desk of Oz, and the Wizard Merlin is off to my right. They are my teachers, my mentors, my friends. From the moment I discovered them between the covers of books, insatiably devouring each word on every page, the concepts and fantasy filled me with the hope of having some power, influence, and control of the fight between good and evil.

In spite of reality messing with my perfect world of idealism, the world that gives comfort in the midst of chaos, I still believe in miracles. I know most emphatically that happiness is within me, in my backyard. Like my dear wizard Merlin, I continue to walk backward in time, with foresight as clear as though new things, thoughts, and feelings have already been. It is my Pollyanna survival.

That time of change in my life and perspective, when death came in spite of every effort to wage war against it, weighed heavily on my shoulders. The laughter in those dark days interspersed with tears. Clouds gathered to darken and dampen the play of sunshine until its warmth became a source of discomfort.

I internalized to escape the changing seasons. I tried to keep constant within myself, lest I succumb to the frailty of the human condition and fall with the autumn leaves, or become barren and cold with winter's sleep. During that time, I stood within myself and stepped out only to give love in spoonfuls to those in pain, to comfort their moments of need, attempting to reach their souls.

My humanity was imperfect, my sanity almost fleeting, but my spirit fought those limitations in an attempt to move about and influence the healing of others. My heart was heavy from knowing the pain and darkness of this world, this life, a sensation I thought was part of maturity, a weight I feared once grasped could never go away. I would imagine that it stemmed from caring for my patients as well as my family members as they fell ill and eventually died. They taught me so much about my past, myself, my place in this world, my spirit's place in the universe. Moreover, in those times, during those lessons, though I thought I was holding the hands of the ill and dying as they passed from this world to the next, it seems they were holding mine as I passed from innocence to understanding and a new spiritual awakening.

It seems that a new day is truly dawning. I am poised in the air at the edge of light as the world remains in darkness. I am above that darkness, aware of it, yet unimpeded by it. My spirit is learning of a plane where I may reside, letting me put into practice all that I have held in theory. It is giving such peace and comfort, and I welcome new knowledge and presence.

Is this characteristic of those who *choose* our types of lifestyles and professions? I have conversations with others in my field who spend a lot of time thinking about death and dying. They have become more aware of the reality of the other side through dealings with those who have gone before. The gift, the knowledge that things may not be so absolute, leads to an enormous amount of speculation and far more questions than answers.

Seeking truth, grasping the lessons of the universe continues, especially as wonders in life and medicine defy explanation. For my patients and my family, I hope through these experiences and introspections to give a higher level of care. I hope to give a level of love that will help and heal in times of pain.

Time changes us all, especially as we deal with situations of grief and loss. I am an eternal child. The love and caring come from the naiveté of that internal child with whom I must never lose touch or banish. Darkness, death, dying, loss – they are backgrounds to highlight and illuminate the positive things that happen. Heartening events are glowing ever brighter in contrast against that darkness.

So forgive me if I seem a little giddy or impudent during my workday as an ER nurse. I may be coping by letting the child within, who possesses far less complex expectations than the adult I have unwillingly become, rule the moment. She gleefully lives in a world of sugar and spice and everything nice, discounting the snips of snails and puppy dog's tails.

~~~

It would seem that medics, nurses, firefighters, cops, and other ES folks are often born with an inherent sense of urgency and responsibility. Whether it is a factor of birth order, heredity, environment, or simply a life choice, some of us seem to have tendencies from our first breath to become rescuers or caregivers. The struggle between innocent child and overwhelmed adult rages within us when doing and seeing things beyond the realm of normal, everyday life. It can haunt us.

The following is a dream full of symbolism from an ES worker who tries to maintain balance and sanity. In our dreams, we sort and try to make sense of what happens during the day, adding in our experiences and upbringing. Some people might say that it's no big deal, but in this story, you will see one adult trying to integrate with the child within.

I have heard that some psychologists try to heal themselves. Perhaps we in ES attempt to do the same. We want to heal wounded puppies, of the two and four-footed varieties so that maybe can heal ourselves.

Remember the four-year-old who wanted to save the dead puppy and eventually save the world? She did not realize until later in life that she first had to save herself. She dealt with those conflicts through her life, painstakingly standing on tiptoes. She carried the cup of responsibility high over her head through troubled waters. She doled out sips of life and breath to others even when she was drowning.

Daddy's Little Girl

I had a dream last night.

When will the memories of childhood be resolved? As an adult, I should be capable of understanding, to explicate the conflicts. They were innumerable years ago, and sleep is my solace, the only freedom I know. Can't there be peace in those few hours? I am not four years old anymore.

Mom was driving a small car, and I was her front-seat passenger. I had a sense of being above the seat, elevated by some entity.

So if I am stuck at being four, let's go with it. If I am ever to understand this child within, and entomb the intrusion of jumping back into her distorted thinking, I have to feel what she is feeling. Perhaps her innocence can remain, and her pain laid to rest.

We were traveling slowly, as though on a pleasant Sunday drive.

Where are we going? Are we moving again? I do not understand, and I am afraid. My siblings are being strong and are not upset, so I have to be that way, too. They are older, so they know better. Is this my fault? Did I do something wrong? Am I not pretty enough, or smart enough? I will be better, Mama. Please just go home and I will be the best little girl in the whole world. I will not even cry... ever.

I was bundled and superficially secure, with a large, wine-colored towel on my lap.

I will sit straight and be still. I will not do anything wrong. Daddy told me I could watch TV if I were perfect, but I was not, and now he is angry with me. It is my fault that he is not here with us.

I was holding coffee in a covered Styrofoam cup, but the sides kept giving in.

This is all just too much for me to handle. I am not like the rest of them, Mama. I am different, but if you find out that I am not good enough, you will stop loving me just as Daddy did. I will make sure you do not find out. It would hurt too much to lose you, too.

I did not understand entrusting a child with an adult responsibility, but the cup was in my hands. The sides of the cup were too soft to hold their shape, so even though the lid remained intact, the external portion would collapse intermittently, and portions of its contents would spill over.

I have so much fear inside of me. If you only knew, it would destroy you, and you have too much to handle already. I will keep it to myself, so you do not have to know about this, too. I can take care of myself. The others need you more than I do. I will be fine as long as you love me, that is all I need, and I will be fine no matter what happens to me.

Not wanting to affect the integrity or appearance of the vehicle adversely, I used the towel, intended for something else, to absorb the hot, potentially damaging liquid.

I am the baby of the family. I can make everybody laugh and smile and take their minds off everything that is bad. No one is in pain when they are smiling and laughing, so my gift to them is to take their minds off the pain and injustice. I can keep them safe.

Having chosen a dark-colored towel to hide the potential staining of the undesired liquid, I made an effort to confine the spillage.

There has to be a safe place to put my fear, where no one can see it. It will not spill over onto anyone else in the family, Mama. They will not have to be stained by the bad part of me, the part that caused Daddy to leave, the part of me that was not strong enough or good enough. I will be the best at everything I do, and you will be proud.

Bounced circuitously with the motion of the vehicle, I struggled to maintain some degree of control.

Why did Daddy hit you, Mama? You were just sitting in the big chair in the living room. He yelled, and he hit you. You did not even move. You looked so small, and I could not help you. I should have been able to stop him when he was hitting you, but I did not know what to do. You did not do anything wrong, and you did not yell or hit back. And if Daddy is bad, why do I still love him? How can you love someone who hurts you, who hurts those you love?

I was trying to balance the coffee to keep it from spilling any more. It was hard to concentrate on what mom was saying and what was going on around me. Keeping the guardianship of the cup with all the intricacies involved in my juggling act was becoming an exhaustive effort. I was so small, so insignificant, not at all suitable for that position, yet wholly incapable of egression.

If I am very, very good, maybe the bad things will just leave me alone. Dear God, please help me through this.

Mom sustained her slow and steady pace, veered slightly to the left and hit the edge of a wheelchair that crossed over to her side of the road. It contained my biological father. Not the young man whose face I knew only from the few pictures I had seen, but Casey, the old man I met in my adulthood.

I sat on the couch, waiting for you, Daddy, but you never came. I stayed there and did not move, afraid I would not be ready when you came to get me for a visit, afraid I might get dirty if I got down, and then you would be unhappy and leave me again. Nonie put me to bed in my clothes, and she was so sad because I would sit there and wait the entire day, hoping you would come to get me, but you never did.

Casey seemed undaunted by the slight jolt, the chrome edge of his wheelchair displaying evidence of previous stressors and impacts from a difficult life.

See Mama? Daddy does not mean to be bad. He cannot help it because he cannot be any better. He does not know how. Maybe his Daddy was bad to him. Maybe he did not have a Mama like you to love and take care of him. Maybe God just made him that way.

I looked up, horrified, powerless at preventing the inevitable. Our vehicle's forward progression was uninterrupted by the impact, moving away from the man in the chair. Through the logic of dreams, he appeared again before us, far enough away to prevent a second collision.

Accepting his fate and our distance, he gave me a smile. In sign language, I said, "I'm sorry" with my left hand, still balancing the coffee with my right hand, still bearing the weight of responsibility. He responded in a sign language that no one but I understood. The words were unclear, muddled by the deformed hands of a man who had experienced three strokes, but I knew he was saying it was OK.

It was not my fault, after all, was it? My Mom and Mike, the Dad who raised me, made me the person I am today. If you, Casey, had been involved in my upbringing, I would have turned out quite differently.

Maybe the darkness and pain, although I learned too soon in life about rejection and loss, instilled the desire to find the light in each situation, in each relationship, in each day. It gave me the desire to make this world a better place. I learned to fight for what is right and good, to work hard because no one will hand me anything that I have not earned.

Each day is a gift that will be as wonderful as I make it. Love is unconditional and truly the greatest gift of all. I thought I was not good enough, but the opposite is true. I am a phenomenal individual with a good heart and a tremendous capacity to give and receive affection. Not everyone in my life is going to abandon me as you did.

It is time for me to grow up, to grow beyond four years old. It is time to be happy with me and put you to rest. Goodbye, Daddy.

Goodbye.

~~~

With thoughts focused on my biological father and the experience of his passing, "Final Directive" spilled out of my fingers. Writing is cathartic. Casey's death had several lessons for me, most revealed in the final paragraphs of the narrative. The role of family member or caregiver ultimately gives us, as emergency workers, greater insight, and empathy when we deal with patients and their families. However, it is a humbling and sometimes scary situation.

Changing roles from provider to family member helps make us better, stronger, and more compassionate toward our patients and their families. It lets us share with them on a different level, allowing bits of self-revelation. Patients and their families sometimes view us as having no personal lives or experiences of pain, loss, or grieving. Saying, "I don't know what you are feeling or how this impacts you, but I've been through something similar," sometimes closes the gap, permitting us to assist at a higher level. Although hard earned, empathy, when sincere, is truly appreciated by our patients and their loved ones.

Final Directive

As I stood by my father's bedside, I found comfort. He had raised his head for me to kiss him, as he always did when I entered the room, and squeezed my hand to let me know he was aware of my presence. He could not answer any of my questions, but I had given up on finding answers long before. Now I was the adult, and he was the helpless child, dependent on me not only for his immediate care but ultimately for the decisions that would end or prolong his life.

The nursing home called at 2:30 a.m. to tell me Casey was not doing well. Awakened from a strange dream when the phone rang, I had hoped the call was just a continuation of those things that your mind attempts to sort out in sleep. The nurse told me that Casey had been refusing his medications and food all day and had stopped responding verbally.

Casey's breathing was very rapid, his heart rate was irregular, and his lab work showed abnormalities. As a nurse, I clicked into an emotionally distancing clinical mode and mentally merged the information given with Casey's medical history during the 20-minute drive to the nursing home. I knew the prognosis was not good.

Casey left our family just before my fifth birthday. I attempted to find him several times, unsuccessfully and without familial support. My siblings were older and had more unpleasant memories than I had, so they bore no desire to find him. Casey was crude at best and his language and conversation not what one might care to share in polite company.

My older sisters had seen him a few times over the years, usually because he wanted to borrow money from them. Regardless of his personality and the fact that he was an alcoholic, I had questions about why he left us, why never visited me, and why he failed to answer my letters. The search became a quest.

Finding Casey after 27 years helped me to realize that the father who raised me, Mike Dudley, was my real dad, and the healing process began. The unresolved conflicts of the abandoned child had directed my decision making poorly my entire life. Through a process of forgiving, healing, and growing, I was finally able to put the childhood pain and abandonment issues aside.

Two of my three siblings still carried their pain and were unwilling to forgive or forget. My sister Nonie, who forgave this very old man, lived thousands of miles away in Arizona. The baby sister was to carry this particular weight alone.

I had checked in at the nursing station before going to Casey's room. The lab work showed elevated BUN and creatinine (kidney failure), elevated potassium (hence the cardiac arrhythmias), and a blood sugar five times the normal level. The nurse had asked before I saw my father, about his *code status*. Were they to intubate or perform CPR? Did I want him hospitalized?

Fortunately, several months before, I had written an extensive and detailed advanced directive and obtained my sibling's legally required signatures. Casey went to the nursing home following a stroke. He was not always lucid and had lost the ability to ambulate or care for himself. Casey's closest living relative was his older brother, Ted, who gratefully accepted my intercessions and explanations the past couple of years.

I referred the staff to that final directive. The directive outlined in detail what to do for Casey in a circumstance where he was unable to make informed decisions. I asked a staff member to call Uncle Ted about his brother's status, and walked to Casey's room.

I thought for a moment about the first time I met Casey when I was an adult. My favorite Auntie, Mary Jo, had located him for me, and we were surprised to know that he lived only 15 minutes from my home. I called him, and we had a superficial conversation. When I asked if I could see him he made several excuses why that was not a good idea, though later he would surely be more prepared.

Having waited so many years and with so many questions in my heart, I ignored Casey's wishes and simply showed up at his front door. I was afraid that he would tell me, "Go home. I told you I wasn't ready to see you yet." He did not. His eyes misted up when he saw me. Without affirmation of my identity, he crossed the room to give me a big hug. His first words were, "You haven't changed a bit."

We went out for coffee that day and talked. He still carried a picture of himself and my mom in his wallet, which made me sad. Here was a man with a terribly swollen liver from alcoholism who lived in one small room. He played cards and watched TV, drinking two ounces of alcohol daily to stay alive.

I vowed that day to see him again, which I did, bringing him playing cards and a painting to liven up the stark walls of his solitary existence. The painting, which I had done in pen and ink and oils, was a flock of birds flying in the bluest sky, freely soaring over beautiful mountains. The picture was such a stark contrast to this man's life and medical condition. I do not think Casey had ever known real freedom a day in his adult life, carrying with him for all those years the demons that shaped his self-imposed prison.

As I reached his room in the nursing home, I realized how small Casey looked. He was only 5'6" in his youth and slight, now withered with illness and age. Here was an old man, maybe 75 (I did not know his date of birth until I got the death certificate after cremation). He had suffered a right-brain stroke with a contorted and atrophied left arm.

Casey's body wandered to one side of the bed due to a loss of the sense we all have of which side is up (proprioception). I moved him back to the center of the bed with a big hug when I visited, so he would not easily notice that I was repositioning him. He always recognized me when I visited, first by my voice, and then by sight.

Sometimes, the residual effects of the stroke affected his emotional state, and he would not be receptive to a visit. He would say things like, "I'm tired. Get the hell out of here and come back another time. They locked me out last night, and I crashed my motorcycle into the building to get back in. Now they won't feed me. Don't come back unless you have hamburgers."

I would kiss him on the top of his head—he always raised his head for a kiss upon my arrival and before departure—and he would look at me with eyes that feared abandonment. He seemed to remember, though he never spoke of it, that he had left an innocent four-year-old child (me), never to return. He would say, each time I left, "You are coming back, right?" At times, he was witty and entertaining, telling funny though occasionally crude stories and often terribly quick with a pun.

Sometimes I stopped in after work, still in a nursing student or paramedic uniform. Casey would introduce me proudly to anyone who happened by. He never mentioned my two siblings who did not want to see him. We talked about my sister Norma (Nonie), and he always asked about my two children, Topher and Missy, whose pictures Casey posted on his room's bulletin board, and whose names he never forgot.

This last time, when I walked into his room, he lifted his head for me to kiss him and squeezed my hand. He mumbled something unintelligible, and I reassured him that everything was going to be fine. Casey took a few drops of water through a straw. He had refused as much from the staff, but kindly allowed me to administer that small comfort.

Rapid respirations and dehydration caused his tongue to furrow and dry. The effort was exhaustive, and he declined any further attempts to drink again. I continued talking without thought of where the one-sided conversation was going, letting him hear my voice and know that I was with him. I wanted him to know that he was not alone, and I would not abandon him.

I looked at him as though he were a stranger. This old man had pasty, thin skin, and a balding head showing scattered patches of wispy white hair. Casey was in the center of the bed, which looked as though made perfectly around him, without even so much as a wrinkle in the white institution-style blankets.

His toes pointed downward, as was the case with most patients who spend most of their lives in bed. The pressure of the linens on their feet curves them down in an unnatural position. When you do not walk, the lower extremities become useless, so they conform to the curve of the blankets as surely as the residents conform to the unnatural lifestyle of a nursing home. Here Casey was with his new family. Three men in a large room who shared the last place they would know as home before passing over to whatever existence their spirits found beyond the limitations of the bodies and building that now encased them all.

Uncle Ted finally arrived with Aunt Mae, whom I knew briefly as a child and did not see again until this day. Ted tried to talk to his brother. Casey mumbled something, and after a few minutes of the three of us staring at him, hoping that he might do something to ease our discomfort, Aunt Mae said we should go somewhere to discuss *the situation*.

In the lobby, we talked about Casey's condition, and I explained his advanced directive. The nurse on duty paged the physician on call. I went to the phone, and the doctor and I discussed lab tests, and whether this situation was reversible, or if were we just delaying the inevitable.

Having seen so many people tell medical staff to do everything possible while hoping for a miracle and needlessly prolonging a patient's pain, I wanted the doctor to be honest with me. I asked if Casey was dying, and if hospitalizing him would simply give him a few more hours or days to die. The doctor assured me that interventions would not correct the situation, and would only prolong the process. Casey was dying. Even if we kept his body alive, he would probably never be back in a way that we knew him.

I explained to Uncle Ted that the best decision under the circumstances was not to ship Casey off to a hospital. IVs and medications would only prolong the expected, death, and to let Casey go. I resented having to be the one to decide to grant or withhold medical treatment and wanted to hand over the gauntlet of responsibility to someone else. I said nothing, of course, but harbored a few thoughts of, "Why me, Lord?" then swallowed those thoughts back with the tears that I refused to let fall. I had to be the strong one, outwardly, even though I felt like jelly inside.

The situation was surreal. I wanted someone to rescue me from having to make life-and-death decisions for my family. It was completely different from handling my patients. I told Ted and Mae I would honor their wishes regarding medical treatment since they had spent an entire lifetime with Casey, but the cup was not to pass. It was my decision. Ted and Mae left, and I went back into Casey's room with a Styrofoam cup filled with coffee and a book.

I always had a book with me. That time it was one of Deepak Chopra's self-help books, which I read to Casey for the next few hours. We had a wonderful one-way discussion of spiritualism and how the very moment we were in was as it should be because the universe was as it should be.

I talked to Casey about Kafka, explaining the hard parts, laughing inwardly for presenting something so foreign to a man of limited education. An unsophisticated man, Casey thought and dealt with things on a simplistic and superficial basis. I told him it was OK to rest because I knew he was very tired and the road and struggle had both been ever so long. I remembered the biblical imperative, "Be still, and know that I am God." (Psalm 46:10)

I watched him closely, waiting for his breathing to ease and then stop, but he continued breathing quite shallowly. I took what vital signs I could obtain every half hour, dutifully recording them on the outside of an alcohol prep pad—my only scrap paper—as though it would make a difference, as if someone might need that information. I watched for Casey's life to end, but he was insistent on hanging on.

Several of the nursing home employees wandered through Casey's room in those hours. They came to say goodbye in their own ways, taunting him to curse at them or tell them, as well, to "Get the hell out of my room, and leave me alone." Funny, isn't it, how people find comfort in unpleasantness just because it is familiar.

Casey responded to no one at that point, not even me. He had stopped mumbling, no longer squeezed my hand, and only moved his eyes slightly in reply to my voice, if that was an intentional response. Nurses wandered in offering me morning coffee and toast. I accepted the coffee, though I do not remember drinking it. It was a normal thing to do in a situation for which one is never quite prepared.

What is the protocol? People can hang on for minutes, hours, or days under these circumstances. No one truly knows when death will come. No one knows what to say or how to behave. Conversations are brief and clumsy, eye contact avoided, and the tension in the air is palpable.

I sat next to his bed, waiting and watching, trying to imprint this image of the person who I had known for such a short time into my memory. I knew he was dying, but dying was an end to things, and I did not have a chance to know if he understood my goodbye. I did not know if I was prepared for this part of my life to end.

In that space between thoughts, I found strength. Freely I sat beside him, not out of obligation or duty, but love. I forgave but had nothing to forgive. The connection between us was not simply biological, but spiritual. The love was God's grace.

It was not for me or anyone else to decide when the time was right or wrong, for the ending of the brief relationship between this biological father and daughter. There is no right or wrong. Things just are, and freedom lies in not judging his life or decisions or when the time for our relationship would end.

I had to leave Casey for a while. It was Sunday morning, and I was in the middle of hosting a two-day seminar on stress management in critical situations. I had the key to unlocking the facility door, a picture that would present itself to me later for greater insight into the day. Only *I* had the key to unlocking the door of understanding.

I kissed Casey on top of the head, said, "I love you, Daddy" and told him I would return. I held onto his right hand for a few moments, feeling the warmth of life still pulsating weakly through transparent flesh. "Good-bye, Daddy."

A memory flashed into mind as I drove to the seminar location. When Casey had first suffered his stroke, I assisted hospital personnel with his daily care. He had said, at one embarrassing moment, "A daughter shouldn't see her father like this." That memory would explain why he held on until after I left his bedside, his gift to me to understand what his death would teach me.

To see an ending to his life would have negated or detained the message of the unending flow of energy, of life. He gave me more in the last five years of his life than in the first five years of mine. From Casey and his death, I gained a gift of understanding, of adding another stepping-stone to my path, to my spiritual walk. In life, though he gave me nothing, in death he gave me everything.

I learned that Sunday that the old explanation of an acorn dying to give life to an oak tree was a fallacy. The acorn does not die. It simply sheds its outer casing to allow for the transference of energy from the shell into the ground and eventually into its new form: the tree. The tree bears the intelligence and experience of that acorn, the tree before it, and finally, the universe that bore them all.

Nothing is lost, and the flow of life continues. The flow of love continues. Everything is as it should be.

~~~

Some emergency services' workers, even though green as a spring sapling, are eager to do what they have seen on TV, and heard about from family members in the business. These newbies grew up with the stories. They have spent time at the station with friends and family, seen tons of gory pictures, and think themselves resilient.

Maybe they are—until something happens that they cannot wrap their heads around. However small the incident, if there is blood, someone may succumb to their emotions and throw professional experience to the wind. To all those who say they are too tough to let anything get to them, I say it just has not happened yet.

We're Not All That Tough

Michele wanted to be an EMT since she was an 8-year-old. Her mother was a super-medic like those on TV. "Mom was the smartest, most competent, best medic that ever lived," or so Michele thought.

Michele took great pleasure in reading Mom's medic books from a very early age, especially fond of the graphic pictures. When Mom went from EMT-Specialist to Paramedic, Michele took the sample tests at home, passing each one. Michele had tons of street smarts and a knack for making complex situations simple, and could find the best alternate when Plan A didn't pan out, just like her Mumma.

Because Mom's greatest skill was starting IVs and Michele had no fear of blood, guts, and gore, she knew that poking holes in people was something she would thoroughly enjoy. Michele also swore that she would do it all without ever spending a day in college. And she did.

Michele graduated from high school and got a job in the same Trauma Center ER that employed her mother. Mom was now an RN, who gained the name *MiM* since *Mom* was not acceptable in the workplace. Mom certainly did not know that Michele pulled MiM from the Magnificent Marvelous Mad Madame MiM, a witch in competition with Merlin in the Disney movie *The Sword in the Stone* (1963).

Michele can handle doing CPR ("I'm getting *such* great abs from it"); flying brain matter (unless it gets on her new shoes); putting her fingers into patient's gunshot wounds, and is famous for getting blood from a rock (obtaining lab samples from people with horrible veins). Old people love her. She is approachable and kind, and treats everyone with the same respect she gave her grandparents, with whom she shared a close relationship. Her coworkers consistently rely upon her; few can work as fast or efficiently, and staff requests her for the hardest duties.

Yep, Michele can handle anything. Well, almost anything. We were soon to find her weakness.

Many of us in ER or EMS often hear, "I don't know how you can do that—I never could." I am not entirely sure that is true. Human beings are more capable than predicted when facing situations we thought untenable, especially when we have no choice, when we *have* to do it.

Some of us are a little more comfortable than the rest of the population, enjoying every minute of the challenges that come with these incredible jobs. We love doing the impossible, making a difference, doing something that would not have happened had we not been there that day, with that person, and in that situation. We can make an indelible impact on someone's life (or death). It is staggeringly satisfying, and as long as we stay somewhat removed from the pain and maintain our professionalism, we can do phenomenal things.

As long as we stay removed ...

MiM had elective plastic surgery (partial facelift and breast reduction) and had to remain in a surgery center overnight on a morphine pump for medical supervision and pain management. Michele was to pick MiM up in the morning after working a twelve-hour midnight shift, which proved demanding and challenging. Multiple CPRs and gunshot wounds translated into no lunch and near physical exhaustion.

When Michele arrived at the surgery center, she seemed unusually distant. Granted, MiM had bandages around her head and arms, with swollen, steri-stripped eyes, arms purple from axillae to fingertips, and stitches from temples to around her ears. One would not expect that appearance to have affected someone who deals with blood and guts every day. Michele could handle bruising and bandages; she saw far worse in her job.

Diverting her eyes from her mother and looking at the cookie sitting on the bedside table, Michele gruffly asked, "You gonna eat that?" and barely waited for an answer before inhaling the cookie. MiM thought Michele was just tired and hungry from the shift, excusing the less than mannerly behavior as she was anxious to get home to bed. The nurse disconnected the morphine pump before Michele's arrival, and the pain of the surgery returned. MiM had already made a trip to the bathroom and back, a marathon for someone who had been through surgery, and was eager to sign out and leave.

Before MiM could say anything, Michele bolted out the door of the recovery room. She asked the nurse just outside, "You got any juice?"

which was also uncharacteristic of this polite young lady. Once again, MiM blamed it on fatigue and hunger but was determined to have a talk with her daughter. When Michele reappeared, the situation dictated that MiM take a different tactic.

"Um, Michele Denise, I think you'd better sit down. NOW!" Fortunately, Michele was accustomed to obeying now and asking questions later. As she sat, Michele, whose face was at best the color of diluted skim milk, said, "Huh? Why? I don't..." and then her head fell forward as she lost consciousness.

Yep. The kid who regularly saw blood, guts, and gore could not handle seeing *her* mom in the same condition as her patients. Mumma was bruised, swollen, and looking as if beaten about the head and arms with a baseball bat (fondly known in EMS and ER as "RTT with a BBB," or "Ratta Tat Tat with a BaseBall Bat").

By the time the nurse came in with the orange juice, Michele was regaining consciousness. She had no idea what had happened. The nurse administered the juice to her second patient and waited a few minutes for Michele to recuperate enough to drive MiM home.

Please know that when it comes to family, friends, or ourselves, we are not that tough. We have the potential to collapse just like you. Michele's co-workers delight in the retelling of that story, hearing how one so strong in spite of her tender years is a total wimp when it comes to family.

I get it. When my teenaged son received stitches in my ER, I slumped over and passed out, too. I had been sitting on the floor next to the gurney where the doctor sutured Topher. Watching with professional interest as the doc repaired my only son's hand, emotion trumped nursing.

I was no better than Michele was at professional distancing. Seeing someone I loved with even a minor wound was overwhelming. The doc just watched me, and when I came to and sat back up, said, "Are you ok?" "Yep," I answered, watching the room still swimming.

And bless his heart; the doc never mentioned it again.

~~~

When working in emergency services, one maintains clinical distance to perform professionally. Compromising that distance can bring the worker to a point of emotional discomfort. When the worker is on the other side of the cot as the patient, the former family of emergency services workers seems cold and uncaring.

The supportive connection is lost, leaving the ES worker turned patient in a place over which he feels he has no control. "Sara" was an EMT deeply into unrecognized caregiver burnout. After giving to others, she had nothing left for herself, least of all love, compassion, or understanding.

Shadows on the Wall

Sara* sat in the dark, watching the moonlit shadows frolic across her living room walls. A warm breeze choreographed the trees' movements as they playfully caressed the silky night sky. She wished to be with them, be one of them, be a part of something bigger and more valuable than herself as she allowed her perceptions of self-worth to diminish.

The darkness became too void of light or hope lately, and her usually strong shoulders began to buckle under the weight of too many expectations. Perfection was a standard that was becoming tiresome and unrewarding, a standard she could no longer impose upon herself, a standard that lost its once shiny attraction as a valued goal to attain or maintain. Too many people wanted a piece of Sara. There was only so much to go around, and with her emotional tank sputtering along on fumes, she picked up the phone and carefully dialed.

"Hi, John. How is life in Bryn Mawr? I just have a quick question, if you have a minute. Does God forgive you for killing yourself? I mean, because you do not have a chance to ask for forgiveness after the fact since you would already be dead. I just want to make sure, I mean, I just wanted to know."

John and Sara had been friends for two years. They met at a church revival meeting, and John was the more spiritually advanced of the two of them. Sara often asked complex questions about her newfound, newborn life because the research (reading the Bible) was not a short study.

Normally, John got back to Sara after consulting with his dad or some other more learned and experienced member of the Oversight, who had spent years studying the document of Christianity. Those folks could cite chapter and verse in answer to almost any inquiry. This last question required an immediate answer, and John was not prepared to give an intelligent response.

"I don't know, Sara. I guess I had never given it much thought. I mean, you are not talking about *you,* are you? This whole situation that you're asking about is completely hypothetical, isn't it?"

Sara felt a pang of guilt at having involved an innocent party in her plan. She wanted this decision and its implementation to be a private affair. Her recent oral surgery provided a full bottle of prescription painkillers, and she had done her homework on the medication's effects.

"No, John. It is not hypothetical. I have a bottle of thirty pills that will assure my stepping over to the other side. I called the poison control hotline and gave them a made-up story about my ex-husband taking the pills from me.

"I told them his height and weight and asked what I should look for as far as symptoms go if he were to ingest the whole bottle. He is heavier than I am, so the effects they described would intensify. I guess I wanted to be sure not to botch it and end up a veggie or gross anyone out by my being found lying in a pool of vomit.

"Anyway, they told me that breathing would become slower and slower until it eventually stopped. Then the heart would stop. It seems all very clean and peaceful, thank you very much. I did not want to tell you, but you are the only person who I can ask about God and stuff.

"So tell me, if I do it, knowing that it is wrong, will God be angry with me? I mean, it's not like I could lose my salvation or anything, could I?"

"You can't lose your salvation, Sara. God's gifts are not returnable. But I do not know if it would be... if it would have any... I cannot say for sure if... I just really need to talk to my dad."

"I don't want you to do that. Please promise me, John that you are not going to tell anyone. They will all find out soon enough, and they will be momentarily surprised, then they will forget all about it and about me.

"They will probably say it was just as well. 'She was not one of us, after all. She's divorced, you know.' Besides, I don't fit. I am not part of your world. Mine just does not make sense anymore, and there is no hope of changing the perspectives of either side.

"I am tired. I am just so very tired. So tell me, does it make a difference or not? To God, I mean. Does it mean that I am not going to be well received in Heaven? I need to know if God forgives an intentionally committed sin."

"Why do it now, Sara? Can't you wait? Besides, I need to know something. I need to know if *you* forgive *me*."

John's anxiety continued to rise as he realized this was not something he could pass along to stronger hands. He was used to reassigning problems to God and waiting patiently for His timing. For some unknown reason, John felt partially responsible for his friend's apparent despondency.

His head swam with thoughts of what he might have done to keep his friend from veering down this very dark and lonely road. He wondered how he could have missed the signs that surely must have been there. As an aspiring preacher, he knew that he was supposed to be sensitive to spiritual needs. How could he have not seen any of this coming?

"Forgive you? Forgive you for what? You have done nothing that warrants forgiving, John. You've been a wonderful friend, and I've enjoyed our times together."

There was a long silence as Sara began to swallow the pills. She was not sure if she should do it daintily, one by one, or just tilt the bottle back and take them all in one gulp. From somewhere, tears began to well up in her eyes and her throat closed a little as she tried to choke them back.

Swallowing the pills all at once was too difficult; she opted for three at a time. What a symbolic gesture, she thought, of the Father, Son, and Holy Spirit. She thought of the spiritual triad, the constitution of man ... thoughts all too abstract and consuming as Sara sought desperately to simplify the weight she carried, and the conflict between spirit and flesh.

"What are you doing?" John feared the answer but asked anyway.

"I'm taking the pills, John. I want to go to sleep and wake up in Heaven. Remember the scriptures? It is a place of 'no more tears, no more crying.' There will be no more pain.

"I can't be what everyone expects me to be *here*. I am human. I thought I could fly until someone told me I could not, and I have been falling ever since. Maybe part of telling you was because I knew you could not stop me. We're pretty far apart and quite frankly, it seemed safe to talk to you since you couldn't intercede."

Sara was right. There was no way for John to stop her. He did not want to let her go, especially since it meant setting her life down, but he had never had to fight before, and he did not know how.

Living with his parents and sister in a fashionable suburb of Philadelphia, John grew up in considerable comfort. Although he worked hard at school, he never wanted for anything. John spent the year between college and graduate school touring Europe, a gift from his father, a respite between goals in an orchestrated professional future.

John owned several dark suits with properly starched white shirts and traditional ties, the accouterments befitting an aspiring architect, and acceptable for his hours in the pulpit as a lay minister. John handled all of his battles on his knees. Beautifully spiritual, but lacking the experience that buys understanding and empathy concerning the suffering of humankind, the reality of the world surrounding his cushioned existence.

John tried to remember if there was anything he could have done differently. Any way he might have been a better friend to Sara. Any way he could have prevented her hopelessness.

He had written her once a month, even sending a pen and ink sketch he rendered of a bridge and peaceful hillside of Wales, knowing Sara had a Welsh grandfather. Sara framed it and told him she would cherish it always. Sara had flown to John's home in Bryn Mawr last winter to ski with a group of young people from the local Gospel Hall, a group that matched her age if not her history. They were all unmarried, and she was divorced with a young child.

Sara realized after that trip that she was indeed different. Although certain kindnesses were extended to her—in the Christian way—Sara's sordid past, being a divorced woman and now single mother, made her ineligible to remarry in their eyes. She wore a scarlet letter, separating her from her peers.

In Pennsylvania, the snow had melted. Although the trip brought to the forefront a painful awareness of a third world, where the newly born-again Christian scorned for past indiscretions must live, she and John had a wonderful visit. Sara promised to come back when John could assure something better than mud-slopes. His past and hers, the differences in their lifestyles and upbringing, and memories of the two years they shared as friends blurred together as John struggled for something to say.

He realized in the depths of his heart how much he had meant to Sara and how their relationship might have taken a different road if she had been acceptable in the Oversight's eyes. Now, facing the harsh reality of humankind outside of his contented and protected world, he had no words. He was as lost in an attempt to guide Sara as she was in trying to find the answers to his questions.

"John, have I ever told you about my front door?" Sara tried to offer John comfort through distraction and possibly hint toward some level of explanation.

"Have you told me about your front door? Is this the appropriate time, I mean, do you really want to talk about your *door?*"

"You should see it, John. It is very old, filled with character if not a little worse for the wear and weather, as with all things in life. Have you ever thought about the symbolism of what a door represents?

"Your perceptions decide whether it is an opportunity or an obstacle. It can be a portal or a gateway to a purpose beyond yourself and your limited concept of time and place. It is the passageway from an area open and seen to an unknown. What lies behind the door is subject to a million variables that change with each moment, adapting to the specifics and influence of each life force that passes by.

"My door leads to a dominion that no one else would understand unless they passed through to experience it themselves. I can assure you that no one would want to walk in my shoes or through my door. Anyway, this door has a diamond-pattern etched in smoked and clear glass. As the moon passes through the night sky, the diamonds change shape and position on the wall. They are my shining stars, set in the night sky that surrounds me.

"I have been watching them tonight, along with the shadows the trees make as they move with the wind. I can make falling stars and wish on them at will. It is sort of like creating your own reality, I suppose. Sometimes, though, the diamonds look like mysterious, unforgiving eyes watching me wherever I go. There's no rest for the wicked, right?"

John had only been half-listening as Sara's words softened to a whisper and slowed with deliberation. He was trying to attract his dad's attention as he passed down the hall by John's bedroom. John grabbed a tablet, and quickly scrawled, "Sara—took pills. What do I do?"

His dad wrote, "Where is she?" and John answered, "Home." As John's dad heavily penciled "Where is home?" John handed over his address book, opened to Sara's name. Dad whispered, "Hang up," and John, offering an excuse about his father wanting to use the phone, quickly complied.

Sara put the phone back in the cradle and finished the bottle of pills. The water tasted bitter as she washed them down, and she found herself surprised that it was not sweet. She had made her decision, and the hardest part was passed. The notes were written, brief and succinct, penned to her loved ones as well as those who would expect them. The flat was clean enough for company.

This world would soon be behind her. This world, with all its tentacles pulling her away from everything that might have been good and worthwhile, would not extract another ounce of flesh. She had sacrificed herself to please humanity and humanity just wiped its feet on her and walked away without as much as a glance back. She gave no more thought to those who she attempted to care for, who simply would not be pleased in spite of her efforts. She let the weight of her perceived failures go and stepped back into the moment.

The shadows on the wall began to dance anew with a rhythmic blue light. Peeking out the window, Sara watched a cruiser quickly come to a halt and park in front of her flat. Two uniformed officers leisurely approached the front porch, saying to each other that it did not look like anyone was home, but somebody filed a complaint, so they had to check it out.

Walking quickly to the back door, Sara slipped outside as the officers knocked loudly on the front screen door. She knew that it would be only seconds before they came in because Sara never locked her doors when she was home. Trusting everyone was one of the reasons she became such an accomplished doormat. Hearing the front door open, Sara jumped the back fence and ran down the alley.

It was amazing how quickly the neighbors, who never knew Sara existed before, suddenly took a great interest in her visitors. Sara walked around the block, standing with the forming crowd of onlookers as a second cruiser arrived. Two officers stood in the front yard talking as the other two checked the backyard, and spoke with a tenant in the upper flat.

"So what's going on?" asked one of the onlookers, to no one in particular.

"I couldn't tell you," responded another, "but those cops came in pretty fast. Maybe it's a drug bust or something. They haven't been in there long."

Sara listened to the theorists and their proposals, occasionally joining in to giggle about how their dull neighborhood was enjoying a few moments of notoriety. These unknowing souls joined because of a fissure in one young woman's life. In a single moment, the seams of her emotional and spiritual being burst apart, and there was no one there to mop up the mess. These neighbors did not know Sara before, did not ask who she was, as she became part of their circle in the night, and did not notice that she was the only one among them not wearing shoes.

Sara walked back down the alley. Hopping over the fence to her backyard was a little more difficult as energy seemed to float almost visibly out of the ends of her fingertips, back into the cosmos. It was not hers to keep, and only loaned for the time she walked this earth.

"There is a balance in the universe," she would always say. "What you put out comes back to you tenfold." Sara had always been the giver, never asking for anything in return, hoping that her gifts would be accepted without anyone chastising her for giving them. Now she prayed for a smooth transition into the next phase of her spiritual walk, wishing not to be rebuked for taking a side step away from her assigned path.

"She's not here."

Sara listened to the officers from her post outside the kitchen window, dumbfounded that these professionals couldn't find a 103# female standing only two feet away from them.

"If people want to kill themselves, *let 'em.* I just wish they would do it and get it over with. It's a lot less paperwork for me, less hassle for everybody else. If people are that crazy, we're better off without them anyway."

The words stung a heart that Sara thought was beyond feeling. Being on the other side of the line drawn between caregiver and client was already difficult, but hearing one of her own declare her as not worth living confirmed her decision and plan as sound. The suffering had become intense, and the pain pills were just beginning to blur the ache of open emotional wounds.

Sara's old coping mechanism, to clinically over-intellectualize, began to fall away with the dulling of the pills. She sat on the flat's back stoop, the weight of her head in her hands, feeling the chill of the night air coldly reminding her that in spite of their declaration of her lack of worth, she was still a part of their humanity. She pitied their deficiency of insight or understanding.

The difference between them and her was very small, in spite of their having reached the conclusion that she was crazy. Sanity is a fleeting thing, and no one who knew Sara would ever have labeled this bright, attractive, energetic and overachieving girl, who had everything going for her, as crazy. Sara dragged herself back inside, curled up on the couch with a familiar old knitted comforter, and phoned John.

"You called the police, didn't you?"

"My dad did, Sara. Don't be mad at me. Do you forgive me? Please, it's very important to me to know that I've been forgiven."

Sara found it strange that she was dying, and the last person she would speak to on this earth was so terribly concerned about forgiveness for *his* sins. This final piece of absurdity failed to mean anything to her. Neither words nor actions had substance and Sara was truly satisfied that the things, people, and considerations of this world were past.

Sara was always an intellectual, a person with a thousand plans running in multiple directions, and eventual successful outcomes. She now wanted to be free from the responsibility of thought, the gift, and skill she used to value as being one of the best parts of her. The last tear fell, and Sara finally took a wonderful, deep breath, feeling it fill her lungs and then exit to the far edge of the horizon, of the universe.

"You're forgiven, John. Now I am going to sleep. I'm tired, and I can't think anymore."

As she fell into the sweetest sleep she had ever known, Sara watched the shadows of trees and diamonds sparkle with life on the walls, inviting her to join them. She reached up toward the dancing shapes as they beckoned, wondering if they were really shadows, or perhaps an apparition of outstretched hands offering forgiveness. To each entreaty, she gratefully accepted.

~~~

Emergency Services workers, whether pre-hospital or ER, will tell you that one of their worst fears is to be on the other side of the gurney. There are folks with degrees and licenses surely purchased on the Internet or awarded from a Crackerjack Box. We clearly have no confidence in those less proficient, especially when our personal experience justly labels them incompetent.

Even if we are fortunate and blessed to be the patient of the most skilled medical personnel, our stress increases with the loss of control. We understand the protocols, treatments, diagnoses, and prognoses. It is at best a scary proposition and quite humbling. This is one medic student's experience of being both caregiver and patient in a single day, facing losing her life, and coming away with a new perspective and worldview. For all those who place people on backboards, may you one day know the joy of riding down a bumpy road on one of those terribly uncomfortable critters yourselves.

Rollover

Maneuvering the old country roads to the hospital, my mind was not on driving. Expecting to spend this New Year's Eve in wonderfully warm Montgomery, Alabama instead of mercilessly cold Michigan, I cursed the EMS instructor. He insisted, at the last minute, on a clinical rotation completion date of 1 January. My son Christopher, a senior in high school, was traveling with his cadet drill team for a national competition at Maxwell Air Force Base.

I hoped to chaperone him instead of spending hours in an ER emptying bedpans. Clinical time is for learning, but if your on-site preceptors are not good teachers, you end up making beds and emptying urinals. You become free labor for the unpleasant tasks the nurses and techs do not care to perform.

As it was less than gently explained to me by one cranky-pants nurse at another hospital, "You have to earn privileges here. We don't just trust people off the street. We had to go to school for four years to do this job, and our licenses are on the line if you make a mistake." Do you think I am going to kill somebody with a too-tight blood pressure cuff, or cause trauma to the patient in respiratory distress by listening to their lungs?

I knew those folks were not going to let me attempt intravenous access (starting IVs), which was the biggest skill I was hoping to practice. The resignation to work the required hours doing menial and not medical tasks tucked into my back pocket as another life experience. I vowed never to repeat that type of attitude should I ever find myself on the other side of the nurse to EMT teaching terminal.

It was dreadfully, bitterly cold. I wondered as I heard the snow crunching under my tires if my son was warm enough (even in Alabama), sleeping enough, eating enough... all the things that go through a mom's mind. Christopher had been a 7-month gestation preemie who I did not get to touch or hold until he was almost a month old. After his birth, while he lay fighting for his life in an incubator, I watched through a window. It was hospital policy to allow only their personnel to touch the critical infants, like my little 3½ pound bundle.

The boy acquired epiglottitis when he was six and almost died. He went into full pulmonary and cardiac arrest with a swollen, cherry red epiglottis that sat like a balloon over his windpipe, cutting off his oxygen. The medical staff performed three rounds of CPR before stabilizing him.

Christopher (Toph) had a significant period without oxygen during the epiglottitis causing minimal brain damage. Later, in private school when tested for aptitude, his IQ was somewhere around 170. I wondered what it was *before* the brain damage.

This kid, who was nicknamed Einstein by his peers, had lapses. Although he learned to handle his personal challenges, this formerly fearless six-year-old boy came home from the hospital with trepidation about even simple things. That he could not even remember to bring his glasses home from school still occupied a corner of my heart.

Toph had become an accomplished musician who sat in first chair in his high school symphonic band, and sixth seat at Interlochen Fine Arts Academy. He achieved third place in a statewide art competition for his first attempt at oil painting. He was a gifted writer. After reading a geometry book one September, he tested out on it successfully in June.

He was a brilliant young man, but I still worried for him and about him. In the midst of those thoughts, memories, and concerns for the boy, who was doing just fine in the Deep South despite my worry, the road seemed to fade away. I felt a mental brain-jolt. My mind's eye saw a flash of something that made no sense. Not a memory, not a vision, not in line with the places my mind had wandered at all.

I drove on, counting down the hours I would spend at this middle-of-nowhere hospital until the completion of my clinical hours. Twice more during the ride into the hospital, I felt the same brain jogging and flashing images that were unidentifiable but familiar, as though a movie was being previewed to me one frame at a time. I dismissed the images, forgot them as I parked the car, and wandered into the ER. Stethoscope in hand, I wore the obligatory and unattractive navy-blue pants and white shirt that labeled me as a pariah (student).

Within a few hours, on this my third consecutive and final day, I was finally assigned to a patient. He was a toddler who weighed barely 20 pounds at 36 months of age. His eyes were vacant and mysterious, sending a chill down my spine.

He should have weighed at least 32 pounds. He should have been playing and running and finding wonder in everything around him, but he did not. He just sat. This child was not eating, not bonding with those around him, not relating to the world or people in a way that was normal or expected.

The boy was not autistic or physically disabled. He was a failure to thrive (FTT) baby. This descriptive term is not a diagnosis but gives information about the child that lets the medical community know, even before examination, that the patient may be severely malnourished and not developing normally, a condition that may be irreversible.

I wondered if the cause was organic (medically based, such as organs of digestion being malformed or incomplete) or inorganic (a psychosocially based disease that may involve poor maternal-child interaction, a psychologically disturbed mother, child neglect, or emotional deprivation). I thought of my children, my beautiful, intelligent, active, healthy, and loving children. My youngest was eight; one continuous giggle, still climbing into mom's lap, a ball of energy, affection, and wonderment since birth.

Christopher and I had also been close when he was small, and people commented that they had never seen a mother and son so devoted to one another. I adored my children, who received and gave affection in great heaps upon everyone with whom they came in contact. My heart ached for this boy, whose name I cannot remember; I tried to distance emotionally from such a sad situation.

I picked him up. He held on to me for several hours, sensing perhaps that this was a mother unlike his own. I selfishly thought about how my arms began to ache. I resented his mother who decided since someone else was holding her child, who was not eating and severely malnourished, that she could go ahead with her girlfriend to McDonald's for lunch. She said she was *starving*.

Mom never came back. I began to come to my own conclusions as to the cause of this boy's illness and figured the unconcerned mother had probably distanced herself from the baby, even before he was born. Remembering when my son was in the hospital so many times in his life, between prematurity, epiglottitis, and chronic asthma, I know that a concerned mother does not leave the child's bedside without good reason. Going to McDonald's because she was "starving" was not, in my estimation, significant or even minimal justification to be away from her very sick child.

Several hours later, the child began to dump, and he was CTD (circling the drain, a slang term indicating that death may be impending). The doctor called for a chopper (medical helicopter transport) to transfer the child to a more appropriate facility with higher levels of care. The child was intubated (a tube down his throat to breathe for him) and prepared for transport. The next hospital's staff would care for him medically, surely remember to stroke his hair, hold his hand, and continue the type of human contact and support that I feared he lacked at home.

When the chopper came, I escorted the boy to the helicopter pad with the doc and nurses. The pad was in the back of the parking lot in a clumsily marked area. A nurse bagged the boy while I, the unskilled laborer, moved the stretcher toward the chopper over ice so slick that each of us almost fell several times.

We took baby steps and held onto the stretcher to keep from falling. The wind was bitter, and the chopper's blades sliced drops of water that formed into ice. The sharp, stinging shards flew toward us, hitting any exposed body parts with noticeable force. I was grateful to have worn long sleeves, and that glasses protected my eyes. I looked around to see those less shielded trying to protect eyes, uncovered arms, and faces.

As the chopper left the helipad, I noticed that I had stayed two hours after the end of my shift. I wondered if my husband had noticed that it was 0100, and I was not home. This was before cell phones.

Even if I had a phone, to call and wake him to say I would be late was unacceptable, as it would have incurred his wrath. I kept my sorrow to myself and got into my car. My mind was beginning to buzz with the memories of the day, how so many pieces of it related to or contrasted with my experiences.

The first 20 minutes of the drive were uneventful. The road was clear, and I was able to hit maximum speeds for the roadways. Tired and emotionally drained, I wanted nothing more than to be home in a warm bed, and to check on the younger child who was home waiting for me. A bright moon lit clear skies, a welcome sight because the farmland lacked streetlights. The darkened homes were one-quarter to one-half mile apart.

The sadness of the toddler's life, situation, and questionable future opened my own heart. I thought about the unhappy state of my marriage, which was also circling the drain, and certainly not long for this world. My relationship with this man who I would divorce a year later had been teeming with unhappiness, emotional malnutrition, and spiritual failure to thrive for many years. The marriage was a mistake from the beginning, entered into under the worst of circumstances. The cause of its certain demise was of no consequence.

I knew that my children and extended family were the only joy in my life. I was suffocating with an emotionally and financially abusive husband who filled every waking moment with strife and conflict. My heart ached for my children, who would leave the home they had come to love. My heart was heavy for all our losses, and the fatigue from trying to continue the pretense of a happy home life was debilitating.

Thinking about these things, feeling physically, emotionally, and spiritually wearier than I ever felt, I hit a patch of black ice. The car began to increase in speed and soon began to spin out of control. Time slowed. Thousands of pictures flashed through my consciousness, as the car spun in circles on the pavement, moving faster and faster after each revolution.

Unable to bring the car back to forward motion, I almost gratefully surrendered to the forces outside myself that had control of my vehicle, and those that had control of my life. I knew the car would stop spinning when it hit something stronger than the car itself, as I knew my unhappy marriage would stop its own out of control spiral only when something stronger took a firm grip and set me on solid ground. I waited.

The car eventually made contact with a part of the road's shoulder that was dry, hitting with such force that the car starting rolling end over end several times. I found out later that had I had hit a light or power pole, I might have been killed, as my model car was weakest at the sides and strongest at the top. I dropped my hands from the steering wheel as I spun, closed my eyes, and tried to relax my muscles. I knew that tightening muscles would cause more pain after the accident should I survive what was certainly going to be a major impact.

As the car rolled, I understood the earlier flashes of images and sensations. I was experiencing them now. The images were of the car losing control, rolling (physical sensations I had never experienced), and landing upside down in a 16-foot partially filled drainage ditch.

There was a sense of calm at this time. An "Aha!" moment. I was not alone. Even though the car and my life were out of control, a force greater than myself was with me. Although I did not think I needed guardian angels, they were there. Spiritual guides who gave me support in the most painful times of my life.

Oddly, I felt comfort and released my life, pain, and future to those forces. I knew they would see to the best outcome. I did not have to fight this or any other battle by myself. I was loved. My heart did not need to break, nor did my body, to escape from the situation that was just another life lesson.

When the car came to a complete stop, it was like when Dorothy finally landed in Oz. The winds that caused her to spin in circles finally ceased and set her into a new place. There was a moment of calm, of wonderment, that the high-speed end-over-end rolling and final landing did not tear my body to pieces. I would later find that I, like Dorothy, landed on the threats to my happiness, and snuffed them out of existence.

Clicking back into clinical mode, I surveyed the immediate situation. Part of EMT training is to do a primary and secondary survey of an accident patient, and my self-IPS (Initial Patient Survey) noted point tenderness in the back of my neck and a sore right ankle. I knew that with neck pain, there could be a fracture.

The best idea to prevent further damage was to remain in the car until help came. It was about 1:15 a.m. on a dark, lonely, country road. No one would be coming. I thought of my children hearing that mom survived a high-speed rollover accident only to freeze to death in her car because no one knew she was missing. After the lights of the car began to dim, while no one came along and the cold began to penetrate my bones, I carefully released the seatbelt and slid to the roof of the car below me.

Looking around the car, I remembered that I had a six-pack of Faygo™ (three bottles each of Red Pop and Rock and Rye). It is a Detroit thing. Those six bottles of frozen pop/soda became missiles as the vehicle sped out of control, rolled through the countryside, and landed upside down in the drainage ditch.

Miraculously, none of the bottles hit me. Five broke on impact, and one of the bottles survived the ordeal, a picture that even the impossible is possible. I totaled the car but kept the surviving bottle of

Faygo as a reminder of the possibility of positive outcomes, even in the most hopeless situations.

The inverted car tilted steeply toward the passenger side, its brand-new exhaust system shining in the moonlight. I considered the possibility of a broken neck, knowing that it was vitally important to keep my head in a straight alignment. If there is a fracture in the cervical spine, movement can cause further damage, including the possibility of severing the spinal cord, causing complete and permanent paralysis from the neck down. It would have made complete sense to follow the path of least resistance and slide out the passenger door.

Something whispered, "No." Not audibly, but in that same sense in which the image flashes came hours before the accident. I followed the direction of that whisper and went uphill, climbing carefully out of the driver's door window.

I found out later that one of the county sheriff 's deputies who came to the accident scene got stuck in the ditch on the passenger side of the car, and had to be pulled out of the partially frozen muck by two very strong policemen. Those officers told me that had I exited the easy way, with gravity through the passenger's side of the car; I would have been stuck and frozen to death before help came. It was another picture for me to say that the path of least resistance is not always the best way. You sometimes have to struggle for the best outcome, but it is worth the fight, and victory erases the sting of battle.

Farmland stretched as far as the eye could see. I carefully turned my body and head as one unit to avoid further injury and evaluated my situation. It was bitter cold, and I was not sure which way to go. That same inner voice, that sense of understanding that I was not alone, seemed to lead me in a particular direction. I followed it, even though there was not enough light to see where I was going. I found a small walkway over the ditch to the roadway in a direction that seemed opposite to logic, in the direction away from the closest home.

Moonlight guided me down the road to a small farmhouse about a quarter-mile away, which seemed to take only a few steps as I walked with a sense of perfect peace. I knocked on the door and told the voice behind it that I had been in an accident and asked if they would please call central dispatch to send an ambulance. The kind elderly couple gently welcomed me into their warm home. Covered in glass splinters, I stood near the doorway to avoid getting debris on their floor.

The ambulance came, and I knew the crewmembers. The attendant in the back who cared for me was, in my estimation, a less than competent EMT. He was one about whom I had joked with other EMTs as being the person who was capable of someday killing someone through his ignorance and negligence. I wondered for just a moment if the angels had left me, if this was a, "Yes, God *does* have a sense of humor" moment.

That EMT, Claude,* put a cervical collar around my neck to protect my C-spine, but it was the wrong size. I could feel that it did not secure my head and neck at all. In spite of that error, or perhaps because of it, I made sure to keep my neck still, knowing the possible complications if I moved my head as we traveled over some very large bumps.

Claude was joking with the paramedic in front who was driving (and supervising Claude) about having *the* Sherry Jones in the back of his ambulance. Claude took several attempts to pass courses and state boards to become a paramedic, and I was always at the top of my classes, a point of contention between us for years. Claude eventually improved his skills to a point of competency and turned out to be a rather nice person once a few years of experience and maturity were under his belt.

Finding the situation rather humorous, he threw the sheet over my head saying, "Here... now you don't have to look at me." I could see the pulse oximeter reading smaller and smaller numbers. Claude did not administer oxygen, which was the standard protocol, and I was watching my oxygen levels get lower and lower, indicating oxygen deprivation. Something in my head said, "Breathe Sherry ... slow deep breaths ... you will get through this."

When I got to the ER, the staff gathered around me saying, "Look ... this is our EMT student." The doctor looked down at me, smelling of oranges from a quick break he had just taken. He smiled warmly and said, "Didn't you just leave here?"

I was embarrassed and uncomfortable about being so out of control, clearly on the wrong side of the gurney. My head ached from being on the wooden backboard, and my muscles were beginning to tense and spasm from the accident. The sensation of broken glass all over me, threatening to cut deeper into flesh than the superficial puncture wounds that I had already suffered, was uncomfortable as the ER staff carefully rolled me onto my side to check my neck and back for pain, injury, or deformity.

Finding tenderness at C 5-7 (the neck) and noting a look of concern in the kind physician's eyes, I knew he was thinking, as I was, of the possibility of fracture. He carefully replaced the collar and said, "Let's keep this on until we get some x-rays, just in case." Somehow, a single tear, whether of pain or gratitude for having survived and finding a kind soul to meet me at the ER door, escaped and began to roll toward my left ear. Knowing that I was trying to be tough and crying was unacceptable, the doctor discreetly wiped the tear away and said, kindly, "I am going to take very good care of you. You made it this far, and the worst part is over; now you can begin to heal."

As the doctor moved down toward my feet, he started untying my shoes to complete the examination. I said, "Oh, please don't do that... I was just here for 14 hours, and my feet stink." The whole room erupted in a relieved laughter, knowing it was a good sign when the patient could joke with them.

Back home, my husband slept soundly. My parents, sleeping on separate floors of their home, met in the kitchen, not knowing why they awoke. They made a pot of coffee and stayed up until I called them at about 0630 the next morning to let them know what happened. I am not sure if my angels woke them, but I know that those who love you connect through something strong, powerful, and enduring. The two people who raised me to be the person that I am knew when I was in danger and were there waiting for my call.

I talked to my dad, told him what happened, and he was in his car on the way to the hospital as soon as he hung up the phone. My dad hated hospitals, but nothing could have kept him from his baby girl. He is the one who drove me home upon release from the hospital.

After a few months of physical therapy, we talked briefly about that night, but dad teared up. The thought of him losing his daughter was too raw and painful to discuss. We dropped the subject and only made brief references to it later. Dad and I were very close, and we often communicated without words.

It is amazing what something like trauma and near tragedy will do. You walk (or are wheeled) away reviewing even minuscule events in your life, and sometimes make a completely new set of decisions and plans. You will either drown in sorrow and impose further self-limitations to your life or grow to take control. After making sense of whatever losses may have occurred, you may realize there is potential for growth.

It is not easy to go from caregiver to patient in a matter of minutes. It is not easy to go from walking a zombie-like existence to taking control and moving forward to accomplish great things with a life spared and given back to you. However, what is worthwhile is usually anything but easy, and certainly worth the effort to achieve.

I hope that what I have done with my life is a testimony to the decisions made that day. I hope that those whose hearts may have been touched realize that pain can be a great motivator. Loss is not always a bad thing as it stirs one to take action. There are still speed bumps, still lessons to learn, but the angels who walked me out of the ditch with a broken neck from an inverted totaled vehicle are holding both my hands today. I sure hope they never let go.

~~~

3	**ER Short Stuff** **The Day-to-Day Life of** **Emergency Room Personnel**

When a patient presents to the Emergency Room's triage desk, one of the first things you ask is their name. The responses can be quite comical, especially when the patient does not know the family member's name, cannot spell it, or has designed a creative pronunciation that often has nothing to do with the letters designated to express that name.

ER Triage: What's in a Name?

RN: May I have the patient's name, please?

Parent: (to patient's older sibling) "Boo, what's your brother's name?"

Parent: "I got it here; it's on this Medicaid card (parent hands triage nurse two pages of names). It's either *this* one or *this* one. Boo, what's your birthday so I can figure out which one is you?"

RN: May I have the patient's name, please?

Parent: "They twins. One is Sean (pronounced Shawn), and the other is Sean (pronounced See-Ann). Their mama named them. Same middle and last name."

RN: May I have the patient's name, please?

Parent: "My baby's name is pronounced, Fa `Ma Lee. Spell it F-e-m-a-l-e." A quick check of patients in the hospital, back when it was not thought to be a breach of patient confidentiality or breaking HIPAA rules, showed that this was not the only "Female" who had been a patient at that particular hospital as there were four others on record.

RN: May I have the patient's name, please?

Patient: "I'm too sick to talk. Ask my husband what my name is ... can't you see I'm sick? What's wrong with you people, asking me questions when it's obvious I can't breathe? You want to know anything; you ask my husband. I don't have enough breath to answer your questions. You supposed to be a NURSE; you should know that."

Patient's Husband: "Her name is Lynette*. Lynette, how you spell your name? And you got it under your last name or my last name or both? Aw, Hell, I don't know, you gotta ask her."

RN: May I have the patient's name, please?

Patient's Mother: "Last name is Smith; the first name is here (on the Medicaid card)." The triage nurse took the card from the mother, put it on her keyboard to enter the information into the computer, and then bit down hard on her lip. The parents spelled the child's name, "Chlamydia." The nurse, Julia, tells me, "I almost peed myself when I saw the name. I had to make an excuse to leave triage before I burst out laughing or wet my pants."

~~~

Creativity is a good thing, but confusion about the proper names for English grammar symbols makes for displaced dashes, haphazard hyphens, abused apostrophes, terminal tildes, and sloppy stroke/slashes. When creating the name for a newborn, we suggest that the parents each have the placement of the symbols indelibly marked on their person, or engraved into something they wear or carry with them. Then, of course, please remember the symbol's name.

I wish I had a dime for every time a mom or dad said, "I know it got some kind of mark in there, but I don't remember where or what it was," which causes multiple registrations for each child. Latoya. Tom. Apple. Good names and easy to remember. I am all for monikers paying tribute to one's heritage. My uncle's middle name was Biaggio, great ethnic name, always caused my spell-check to alert that it *may* be a misspelling. Good thing it was not `Bi'Ag-gio~.

~~~

Sometimes not having a name to associate with a patient can cause great delays in communication with family members, and possibly inappropriate care and treatment of patients. As I write this, I am sitting in my hotel room at the Ritz-Carlton Cancun looking at the waves crashing lazily onto the beach. I do not have phone service here, but my iPhone stays with me because it contains my emergency contacts, insurance information, medical history, medications, allergies, and most importantly, *who I am.*

Last night we were on our way back from a company dinner. We were with about 100 other folks employed by, or distributer's for, a large company for which my husband sits on the board of directors. A young adult female got onto our transport bus yelling, "Mom. Mom. MOM! Take my purse!" The young woman tossed the purse to her mother and gleefully left the bus on her way to an evening of what one might assume to be fun and frolicking.

I looked at my husband and said, "Without identification? She is going out at night to party in a foreign country with no ID on her at all?" Ed, sitting in front of us, said, "She probably isn't going to pay for a drink all night so that she won't need her purse." Logical, I suppose, but ... what if something happens?

What came to my mind immediately was the day a young male Hispanic came into our ER resuscitation room in full cardiac arrest. He was obviously in good health (before this day), transported to us via EMS from a fitness center where he had been running on a treadmill. He dropped to the floor without any prior notice that something was wrong.

While the staff was waiting for EMS to arrive, they gathered a handful of ID cards that *could* have been this young man from a stack at the front desk. It seems their policy was to collect the ID of each person as they checked in to use the facilities. Staff returned ID cards to members as they checked out for the day.

We received six ID cards, all with pictures of young Hispanic males, any of whom could have been our patient. A few of the nurses were discussing, after they called the code and pronounced the young man dead, whether they should call the family of the person the fitness center ID card most likely resembled. My head spun around a few times before screeching to a halt.

What if NONE of the ID cards presented belonged to this man? What if we guessed incorrectly and told folks their family member had just died? "Oops. Sorry. Guess it was not Jose*, it was Guillermo*. My bad."

We waited for the police to arrive. The officers could work toward positively identifying the body before shipping it to the morgue for autopsy. Nevertheless, the fact remains that there was no identification. Lesson learned is that I would sincerely advise all of you and your family members to carry some identification on your person at all times. If medical conditions exist, please outline them in some way (ICE on your phone or a paper list in your wallet). More than the absurdity of name spellings and pronunciations is the fact that not having identification and medical information can cause a delay in appropriate treatment or family contact.

Do not wait for a toe tag.

~~~

When a patient approaches the ER triage desk, we ask, "What brought you here" or "Why are you here today?" When the answer is "the ambulance" or "my brother," a clarifying question follows, such as, "How can we help you today?" Simple questions. Here are some of the not always simple responses.

ER Triage: How Can We Help You Today?

Patient: "I'm having chest pain. You gotta take me first; I'm not waiting behind all these people when I could be having a heart attack."

Nurse: "Ok, you are 22, no medical history, taking no medications, no one in your family has ever had heart problems, and it hurts more when you move, or when you press on it, and you've been lifting weights, which is new for you. You originally told me that you were here because you dropped the weights on your foot (that you are easily walking on), and you wanted to make sure that the foot was not broken. Now you want to go in front of all these nice people, who are very ill, and got here long before you because you suddenly have chest pain. Sir, your risk stratification is low, your vitals are completely stable, and you will have to wait your turn. I apologize for the delay; please have a seat."

Patient: "Fine. Then I'm going outside to smoke. What happens if I drop dead out there?"

Nurse: "Well then sir, you'll move right to the front of the line."

~~~

Patient's mother: Mom came to the triage desk stating that her infant twin boys were suffering runny noses, and she was sure they had (both) stopped breathing several times. The babies, about six weeks old and breathing just fine, did, in fact, have dried matter around their noses. When asked, mom stated she did not clean any of the debris off their faces because she wanted to prove to the ER staff that it existed.

Grandma chimed in that she had done CPR on the babies to save them. All family members needed copious amounts of education. Discharge papers included several pages of written instructions for follow-up, and the babies, perfectly healthy except for slight runny noses, went home.

~~~

Patient: (slumped in a wheelchair and speaking in a whisper, gasping between words) "I can't stand this pain. My chest. It feels like the muscles are being pulled out from the inside."

After determining that the complaint was not a result of cardiac problems or injury, the nurse was able to get the patient to pinpoint the day, almost a week ago, when the pain started. He said he must have "rolled over hard in bed" to cause such agony. He also admitted to smoking medical marijuana to control the excruciating pain.

Like so many others who sometimes dramatize their complaints for effectiveness, this patient, who could barely talk or move in the chair during his triage, got up and walked effortlessly to the waiting room when his triaging was complete. Were it not for HIPAA, I have often thought we should film the patients to compare and contrast patient activity and breathing when the nurse is looking, and when the patients think the staff is out of sight or earshot. It can be quite the show. Some might even find themselves up for an Oscar, Emmy, or at the very least a candidate for winning the $10,000 prize on America's Funniest Home Videos.

~~~

Patient: "I want me and my four kids checked out. We were in a car accident. Some idiot bumped us from behind at a stoplight."

Nurse: "Was anyone hurt?"

Patient: "No, but you can never tell. They all look fine, but I want x-rays from head to toe to make sure they are ok. I'm gonna sue if they ain't ok, so I want it all documented."

~~~

Patient: "I'm here for a pregnancy test. I don't want to use the ones at the store because yours are better."

Nurse: "Ma'am, we use the same ones that you get in the store, we just buy them in bulk. If you have no medical complaint or concern, you *can* just go to the store and buy one for a few dollars. The emergency visit is going to cost you close to a thousand dollars."

Patient: "Yeah, but I don't have no insurance, so I'm not paying for this, and if I go to the store they make me pay. Sign me in for my free pregnancy test."

Some young women reproduce and then assign names to their offspring that they can neither spell nor remember. Something they have made up because it sounds so cool and unique. Characteristically, they often do not have a clear idea regarding the child's paternity.

Do we as ER nurses become a bit acerbic when faced with this same situation day after day, week after week, month after month? Of course, we do. Despite our efforts to maintain a professional distance, we are still, in many cases, parents ourselves. Particularly sad is that the young girls coming in for their *free pregnancy test* are often in their early teens.

~~~

Patient: (delivered by EMS naked, dirty and covered with a blanket) "My boyfriend left me at the bar in the middle of a mud puddle." Not much I can add to that.

~~~

Patient: (27-year-old female) "I'm having vaginal bleeding and cramping today."
Nurse: "When was the first day of your last normal menstrual period?"
Patient: "About a month ago."
Nurse: "Congratulations, you're having your period."

Patient: (Nervously, to triage nurse, after being told the nurse would be taking the patient's vital signs, which consist of the measurement of temperature, pulse, respirations and blood pressure) "Vital signs? I have VITAL SIGNS?"
Nurse: "Geez, I sure hope so."

~~~

Patient: "What brought me here? The ambulance brought me here. You don't see these guys in uniforms standing right here? You people got me worried."

~~~

RN: "Nursing is toxic."
By way of explanation, Jim relayed a story that is typical for an ER nurse but not normal experience or conversation for the average person. He tells me that while working in triage, he had an all too common complaint by the patient of having a foreign object stuck in their rectum. Apparently, this male had taped the working end of an electric razor to avoid injury, and desiring the effect of vibration, had inserted the square razor into his rectum.

When the patient tried to pull the cord to remove the razor, the cord detached. The razor worked cordlessly. Jim says they sent this patient to surgery and remarked that "There are much cheaper ways to get a prostatic massage."

~~~

Patient: "I'm here for the same thing I was here for last time. You have it on your computer. I'm not telling you again. I don't have the time to keep repeating myself, and I can't be expected to remember all of my medications, which you goddamned people insist upon asking me every time I come here. Look it up."

~~~

Patient: "I'm out of my pain medication. I have chronic back pain, and there is nothing anybody can do for it. I want Vicodin 10mg, don't try to give me the 5mg, it doesn't work.

"And can I have some Valium with that to help the back spasms? They've done all the tests. I don't need any of that. I've got a copy of my MRI in the car if you need to see it. Just give me a refill for my prescriptions."

~~~

Patient: "I had five seizures today. I stopped taking my medicine because it was New Year's and I wanted to be able to have some champagne."

Patients on seizure medications commonly stop those medications when they desire to drink alcohol. The patient had another seizure in his wheelchair at the triage desk, and staff rolled him into the resuscitation room for treatment. Good thing he did not seize while driving to the hospital and kill himself or somebody else.

~~~

Patient: The man, thrashing in his wheelchair and throwing himself on the floor due to "excruciating pain," was noticed by the charge nurse and put into one of the gurneys designated for patient EKGs) "I have kidney stones. I've had them before, so you have to give me Dilaudid right now." The patient continued to thrash on the bed without exhibiting any medical indications of difficulty in his vital signs.

There was no blood in his urine, and the nurse had risk stratified him to be of very low priority. The triage nurse was not happy with having to take on the responsibility of this patient's care while trying to triage 30 other patients waiting in the lobby. She asked a certain doctor, whom she knew did not put up with overt drama, to evaluate the patient.

The doctor, who also held a doctorate in pharmacology, did an expert evaluation of the patient and gave the nurse the type of order she had never before received: "Give the patient Dolobid (an anti-steroidal, anti-inflammatory, non-narcotic, pain medication pronounced DOUGH-low-bid) and pronounce it Da-LAW-bid when you give it." The idea was that the patient would think, perhaps, that he was getting the narcotic Dilaudid (pronounced Da-LAW-did). With the medication given as ordered, the patient was soon happy.

Another physician ordered a sound-alike medication some years ago on an interventional cardiology unit. I was newly into nursing and did not think it was ethical to misrepresent medications to the patient, but there was enough Paramedic in me to try it. The patient was complaining of pain after a cardiac catheterization. The test was clean (no problems identified), and the patient was staying overnight so we could watch the puncture site. This was years ago when patients had to lay flat for eight hours to prevent poke holes in the arteries from losing their clot/patch and re-bleeding.

This patient was not getting pain relief from anything we gave him. He insisted that he needed more morphine, and was becoming increasingly agitated. I called the house doctor repeatedly to the bedside, a doctor who refused to give the requested medication. Finally, the House Officer, or HO as we affectionately called them, pulled me aside and gave me a very specific order, which I was not to write into the patient's chart.

The HO had told me, in front of the patient, "I want 4 mg NS IV Push. That should take care of the pain." When we were out of earshot of the patient, the HO smiled and said, "Yes, I said 4 mg NS. Normal Saline. Let me know how it works."

Inside the medication room, I pulled up 4ml of normal saline. NS sounds like MS, which doctors used to say for Morphine Sulfate. I marked the syringe with a red sticker noting the name and dosage of the med, date, time, my initials, and date of expiration, as we did with narcotic administration.

I walked into the room and told the patient he was getting the 4mg of NS that the doctor ordered, and went through the steps one would use in giving a narcotic. I wiped the port with alcohol, pinched off the tubing and slowly administered the NS following it with a flush of normal saline to make sure the patient got the full dosage of medication. I heard nothing more from the man until the next morning when he said, "Thanks for being so understanding and staying on that doctor until he gave me something that would help. That is the best night's sleep I've ever had."

Who said placebos do not work?

~~~

Patient: "I've been having trouble breathing (or: swelling in my ankles, headache, arthritis, abdominal pain, can't keep anything down, diarrhea, chest pain, spasms in my legs, my mouth waters, my eye is twitching) for six months (to 10 years)."

Nurse: "What is different about it *today* that brings you to the Emergency Room *today*?"

Patient: "I couldn't take it anymore. This is Saturday, and I don't have an appointment until Monday with my doctor (who has been treating me for all these complaints for the last six months to 10 years).

Nurse: "The emergency room treats and stabilizes new conditions; may I ask what you expect from your visit today?"

Patient: "Well, you people gotta know more than that doctor if he couldn't figure out what was wrong in 6 months (to 10 years). I want you to fix this NOW, and I'm not going home until you do."

~~~

Patient: "Well, this is pretty embarrassing, but my wife and I were experimenting, and I think her vibrator is stuck in my rectum." X-rays confirmed that this 21-year-old heterosexual male had indeed lost a vibrator after insertion into his rectum—backward. The battery pack was toward his umbilicus (belly button).

The batteries had long since worn out, but the man was unable to remove the sex toy, or have a bowel movement. After three days, he was suffering excruciating abdominal pain. Surgery was successful, and the young man made a complete recovery.

Stories about foreign objects in the rectum are common. Consider this a public service announcement if you know anyone who likes to experiment. These situations can be life-threatening, and sometimes require major surgery followed by a long and painful recovery. I always wonder, though, how the insurance company deals with paying for the hospitalization, or what the patient says to his coworkers to explain his prolonged absence.

~~~

Patient (Male): "I'll tell the doctor. It's too embarrassing to tell you.

Nurse (Female): "Sir, I'm afraid if you don't tell me something, I cannot make a chart, and without a chart, you cannot get into the back to see the doctor to get treatment."

Patient: "Ok, I have a runny nose."

Something was running all right, but it was not his nose, as usual with males too embarrassed to give the *real* reason they came to an inner city ER for treatment. The patient got a painful and powerful shot in the bum (buttocks), and some oral antibiotics following a urethral culture, which is a giant Q-tip down the penis. The young man had seen a female triage nurse, female doctor, and another female nurse to treat his sexually transmitted disease. Some days you are just not dealt the best cards.

~~~

Patient: (40-year-old male) "I've got a Depends™ partway stuck up my butt."

Nurse: "How did it get there?"

Patient: "I have no idea."

~~~

Patient: "I feel like my female parts are going to fall out."

The triage nurse contemplated multiple strategies and comments, but resisted verbalizing them, or handing the patient a plastic basin to catch said parts, in the event she realized her worst fears.

~~~

Nurse (to her coworkers): "I'm sweating, and I stink."

Sharing comments that one would not necessarily divulge in polite company is normal for ER staff. Announcing that one is "going to pee" is necessary so someone can listen for your patients, for example. This nurse, who was running the first four hours into her 12-hour shift, breezed by the secretary's desk, and unceremoniously made that announcement to anyone within earshot. Apparently, things did not improve much as she felt the need to share, several hours later, "I'm still sweating, and I smell even worse."

Whatever happened to "Hello?"

~~~

Nurse: Walking quickly from triage to the patient care area, Peter, my all-time favorite and clearly the most brilliant RN ever known to humankind, stopped suddenly and exclaimed, "Ooh... Brain Fart ... smell it?" Sometimes those things catch you SO off guard that you can feel the rubber band in your head pull taught and snap. It can cause serious brain damage.

~~~

Nurse: "I didn't touch a thing. I want a witness. Four *empty* 100mg vials of Demerol just fell out of the patient's pocket. Can you give me a hand in here?" Several patients, as well as staff, heard her, so there were enough witnesses to back up her position and provide documentation.

Just before that statement by the ER nurse, Debbie,* two other nurses had escorted a staff nurse from the floor down to the ER. They thought she was having a stroke. The nurse/patient was slurring her words and had an unsteady, shuffling gait. She could not walk under her power.

Debbie had assisted the patient behind the curtain and helped her undress. As the patient removed her lab coat, there was a tinkling sound heard from behind the curtain. Hearing the sound, another nurse peeked behind the curtain as Debbie backed away and out of the curtained area with her hands in the air. Several narcotic vials were on the floor, one rolling out from under the curtain in front of other staff members, patients, and patients' family members.

The floor nurse had been sharing her patient's prescribed pain medications ("a little for you, more for me"). We called security and the nurse/patient, who was not having a stroke, but was high on Demerol, followed her hospital stay with a trip to rehab. She eventually returned to duty without losing her license, which is the norm for this type of circumstance. I hope I am never on the other side of *her* gurney.

~~~

Triage nurse: "Can somebody help me in here? I've fallen, and I swear this isn't funny, but I can't freaking get up."

Julia, the same Julia who ran out of the triage area to keep from laughing at the child named Chlamydia, had been triaging a sick child. Julia slipped in a pool of the child's vomit on the floor. With a badly broken arm from the fall, we thought Julia would gain some well-deserved time off. We, who tire of the ruthless and unforgiving pace, often look forward to things like minor surgeries and illnesses because it means time off work. We rest, recoup, and recover, regaining our zest for our chosen careers.

No such luck. With a fractured and casted arm, Julia was incapable of performing nursing tasks requiring two hands. With one arm in a sling, she was unable to bandage, start IVs, administer medications, etc. Julia's reward was a permanent assignment: she would spend the next four months at the same triage desk where she broke her arm.

~~~

Patient: (Gagging between words, while bending over a large bucket with her fingers down her throat) "I'm here because I'm throwing up."

Nurse: "Ma'am, please don't do that. If you stop doing that (putting your fingers down your throat) you will stop throwing up."

~~~

Posted on the employee bulletin board are several comments from patients. This one started out as a monolog about a patient's long wait in triage. The best part is the employee comment at the end.

Patient: "I spent four hours waiting for a doctor to show up for less than three minutes of care. The staff stood around behind the desk doing nothing. They felt my condition only warranted a gurney across from a bathroom. How do I get a job that pays well to do nothing?"

Staff: "Go to school."

~~~

A patient came by wheelchair to triage from the cafeteria, where she had been helping herself to food without paying. As she was an ER patient who left before discharge, she was still wearing a hospital gown. The patient stated to hospital staff that she needed to see a psychiatrist.

Psychiatric complaints are always a good way to get out of paying for lunch. The woman denied homicidal or suicidal ideations, meaning she did not intend to hurt herself or anyone else. There was no urgency to rush the patient back to see the physician, who was about to discharge her a short time before. The patient's name was put back into the system, and she was placed in the lobby just outside the triage desk.

Once a patient leaves the ER, staff must create a new visit chart, starting a new paper trail. The patient grew impatient and agitated, knocking over the floor-mounted hospital signs. She yelled, "You have to see me right now. I need Haldol" (an anti-psychotic medication).

The patient was brought into the triage area where an ER tech took her vital signs and documented on her chart pertinent data such as medications, medical and surgical history, and allergies. I removed the patient's large bag of belongings and placed them safely out of reach. Then I called around the ER to find a bed for her.

One of the nurses who answered the phone said she "just got rid of that loud and belligerent" patient, and refused to see her again. The patient was about to be discharged when she wandered off to the cafeteria. "I'll send Dr. W. out there to finish her paperwork."

While I was speaking with the nurse, the tech, for reasons I still cannot fathom, gave the patient back her bag of belongings. Dr. W, who had seen the patient in the ER, came out to triage to continue her discharge instructions. Dr. W said he was not going to write her a prescription for the narcotic pain medications she was requesting (demanding), and that she should follow up with her doctor.

Before the doc could finish his instructions, the patient reached into her bag and pulled out an iron (the kind used to press clothing), jamming the point of it into Dr. W's head. I heard the patient yelling and Dr. W saying, "Call Security, she stabbed me." I flipped the panic switch. We do have them, though rendered somewhat ineffective when staff, instead of responding to the emergency, floods the phone lines with calls asking, "Is it a real emergency?"

There was blood everywhere. Dr. W was holding a compress to his head to stop the bleeding that had quickly obliterated his features. Security separated the woman from the weapon. This time, there would be no apologies, or fruit baskets, for a patient not happy with the service.

Detroit's finest came to take the woman away in handcuffs. The physician levied charges against her. It is sometimes a war zone in the ER, and staff members do get hurt, sometimes quite badly. Wish they would bring back Hazard Pay.

~~~

Triage ER Tech: (on the telephone) "Momma if you are watching the news, and you hear anything, I want you to know I'm ok."

My daughter worked in a Detroit city trauma center, and I was doing crisis-management work at Maxwell Air Force Base in Alabama. Far from home, and incapable of protecting her or coming to her aid, I took a deep breath. She began offering an explanation.

"Well, there was a guy who came in, and before he even got to the metal detectors, he shot up the ER entry. The security guys pulled their guns and shot him. He didn't hit any of us, but I think he killed the guy in front of him."

The walk-through metal detector sat next to the door where the techs picked up wheelchairs and discharged patients. It was not secure, and that gunman could have killed any of our techs, nurses, or patients. By God's grace, our staff and patients escaped injury.

The hospital representative held a press conference with local television reporters. "No staff members or patients were ever in any danger." I wondered what she had been smoking.

I am hoping that my daughter will go back to college and find a safe desk job somewhere.

~~~

When a patient-separating curtain appears solid and sound defying, people standing nearby often overhear things not intended for sharing. The results can be embarrassing for some, delightfully comical for others. When I started teaching CISM classes and doing public speaking, I explained to audiences that I trained my voice to stay within a certain distance to avoid embarrassing patients who had nothing between them and the world but a few feet of air and a cotton curtain. Perhaps this section will help folks understand why a lowered voice is good for maintaining privacy and dignity.

A Curtain is Not a Wall: Things overheard...

"Ma'am, you walked in here under your own power, I'm not going to lift you now because you're in bed. Besides, look at me. I weigh 125 soaking wet, and you are more than 300 pounds!"

~~~

(To a patient who suddenly and without explanation loses the ability to reach her bottom after having a bowel movement) "Who wipes your butt at home?"

~~~

(To the patient who sees an opportunity for drama and attention by putting his head through the bars of the gurney, and fakes seizure-like activity) "Get your head out from between the bars, sir, and please stop spitting. That is NOT human behavior!"

~~~

(To the homeless patient, who is completely alert and oriented, but decides it is too much trouble to step 50 feet to a bathroom; he steps gingerly out of the clean, warm gurney, and takes aim at the corner of the room) "Sir, the wall is not a urinal. Would you like a urinal? Sir... you are splashing urine all over the place. Sir, please stop urinating on the wall. Sir!"

~~~

"Mr. Brown,* I cannot find your penis. When is the last time you saw it?"

When male patients become obese, very often their penis will retract and become difficult to locate. A nurse trying to place a Foley/Urinary catheter in a 500-pound male uttered those words in frustration.

Unsuccessful at placing the urinary catheter herself, the nurse began strategizing with the doctor and two ER techs just outside the patient's room. They were near enough the nurse's station to be overheard: "Ok, we'll stand him up, you two hold his apron (belly) with sheets, and one of us will go in with the Foley catheter. So... who has the longest arms?" The doc, who unfortunately had a short nurse and shorter paramedic working with her that day, found that when the three compared wingspans, she lost.

~~~

Patient: (snapping her fingers at the nurse): "I want a warm blanket and a pillow... and get me some food; I ain't had nothing to eat in a week."

The nurse explained to the patient that medical care would be the first consideration. She could not have anything to eat or drink since her complaint was of nausea, vomiting, and abdominal pain. The patient shot back, "You are here to take care of all my needs. If you don't get me what I want, you get me the nursing supervisor. NOW!"

Sometimes I wonder if there is a sign at the front door: "If you don't get what you want immediately, regardless of whether or not it is in your best interest medically, please demand a nursing supervisor to complain about the staff and you will probably get something *free*." The patient did, in fact, get a small basket of candy bars and goodies from the gift shop. I am sure she went home and told all of her friends how to get free stuff from the ER by belittling the ER staff and making unreasonable demands. Squeaky wheel ...

~~~

(MD to patient, who was dictating to the doctor what tests to order, which tests he did not need, what medications he wanted, and in what dosage): "I'm sorry pal, but you aren't ordering off an a la carte menu."

~~~

Patient: (physically healthy young female in a corner bed who felt the staff could not see her from the nurse's desk): "ExCUSEme, I'm having a cardiac arrest over here. Can you hear me? My heart stopped. Is anybody gonna do CPR on me? Hell-ooooooo!"

~~~

Patient: "I heard what you said, and what that nurse said, and you are discriminating against me."

MD: (evaluating a 450-pound woman loudly complaining about the medical care she received thus far, and the comments she overheard when rounding outgoing staff gave report to incoming staff):

"I'm sorry to hear you feel that way, ma'am. Would you like to tell me what happened?"

Patient: "That nurse said I was morbidly obese. You people got no right to make judgments like that. You're supposed to be professionals, not calling people names, and telling me I'm gross."

MD: "Ma'am, being described as morbidly obese or grossly overweight are medical terms. They are not social comments. I'm sorry your feelings were hurt."

Patient: "Well, then, do I get a fruit basket or something because you offended me?"

~~~

MD: (giving discharge instructions to a very large woman, and using a *very* thick Asian accent): "Ma'am, you can't breathe because you too fat. You go home, lose weight and then you can breathe. You too fat to breathe."

The patient nodded, thanked the doctor, and took her prescriptions, promising to do better. Apparently, an accent and perception of English as a second language is not as offensive as clear-speaking Americans. Best part of this story is that the doctor was born and raised in Detroit.

~~~

MD: Dr. Doug Wheaton is a very buff, brilliant, ER doc who stands up for his staff. He will not allow them to be abused by patients who come in drug seeking, wearing a giant chip on their shoulders, or carrying a sign that reads, "The world owes me." I wish I could tell you what Dr. Wheaton said to those patients who were verbally (and sometimes physically) abusive to his staff.

Dr. Wheaton always pulled the curtain and then whispered in the patient's ear. When Dr. Wheaton then pulled the curtain open and exited the area, the nurses never had another problem with those patients. We always wanted to know what Doug had said to them, but that remains one of the world's greatest mysteries.

Dr. Douglas Wheaton, we love you for watching out for us. Instead of doling out Demerol and Dilaudid to whoever asked for it in the quantities they specified, while making the nurse apologize for the sins of the entire world in that patient's long and sordid history, you stood your ground. You are the best, and if there is a follow-up to this book, perhaps you will share some of those conversations. I will change your name. No one will ever know it was you.

~~~

RN to MD: (Conversation overheard while the physician was suturing a patient: The doc wanted to know if the RN caught the latest political news on the television.) "Oh, no... I don't watch the news unless I have to. My husband has it on all the time, so I do catch some things, but for the most part, we get enough bad news and life-and-death stuff at work."

It is true. Many of us may keep up with current events through the internet or newspapers. However, several of us do not watch the news on TV except for perhaps the satirical editions. It is too depressing to spend all day making life and death decisions and then go home to see all the sadness of the world. We want to put that behind us for the twelve hours of solace we enjoy until we go back to work.

ER Nurses are often overly cautious moms, too. The *what ifs* in life are daily realities, so ignoring the possibilities of their occurrence is not a choice for us. Our children can tell you that we are extra careful, and think of things other moms cannot fathom as we send our kids out for the day with specific warnings about what is *out there*.

Some of us live in anticipatory grief, knowing that there is no safe place, and loss of health, life, or limb is a reality we cannot ignore. We carry that silent weight, that unidentifiable feeling in the pit of our stomachs, and do not often express or admit it, even to ourselves. We almost envy those who live life in abandon ignoring the possibility of what if, but at least we are somewhat prepared. For me, when the bad news comes, and it always does, I can safely say that the last words I expressed to those closest to me were, "I love you."

~~~

EMT: I love to listen to Kitty,* an ER tech (ERT) when she is with patients. They love her, especially the older women, who Kitty always treats with the same care she gives her grandmother. Kitty has a quick wit, enjoys her job, and has always wanted to be an EMT.

One day, behind the curtain that patients (and sometimes staff) think is a soundproofed wall, I heard Kitty dealing with a patient who was obviously hard-of-hearing. The patient needed to drink Barium for an upcoming X-ray. The woman was confused and needed lots of prompting.

For those who entered the room and were not aware of what was going on behind the curtain, there was a surprise in hearing Kitty tell the patient, quite loudly, "No, Honey, SUCK it. SUCK IT. There you go. GOOD GIRL!" When Kitty threw back the curtain, several staff members winking and grinning greeted her. Only then did Kitty realize how her direction *might* have sounded to the untrained ear.

~~~

ERT: A 50-year-old female patient came into the ER complaining of flu-like symptoms, wrapped in her comforter from home. Lacking a call light to summon staff, the patient yelled through the curtain. "I need a nurse in here. I crapped all over myself, and you need to clean me up."

The ER tech said she would be happy to walk the patient to the bathroom where she could clean herself, but the patient declined. "No, I'm sick, *you* gotta clean me up." Twenty minutes later, the patient left with discharge instructions, washcloth, soap, and a towel.

~~~

Patient: "Jesus Christ, you f—ing people really piss me off."

What was the reason for the patient yelling expletives at the nurse? The patient said she had a terrible migraine and was too weak to walk to the bathroom, which was about 10 feet from the end of her bed. The nurse offered the patient a wheelchair or a bedpan, but it would have been far more dramatic for the patient to lean on a nurse and possibly have her knees buckle in front of a crowd for the sympathy vote. Angered at not having her desires met, the patient stomped to the bathroom under her own power with a very steady gait. Seems she did not need help after all.

~~~

Patient: "F— you, f— ing doctor and nurse. Get your trashy, punk ass out of here, bitch. You and your evil a—hole, you bitch, I'll meet your ass outside when you get off work. You better be careful when you go out the door. I'll meet you in the parking lot."

Obviously, security escorted the staff member to the parking lot after work. Threats to ER staff are all too common. You will see that most of us have a name badge noting only our first name and last initial.

It makes me wonder about the staff doctors who use their full names. Are we not concerned about their safety? On the other hand, perhaps we have not evolved to the point where nursing staff deserves the same respect. We should be saying, "Dr. Jones,* meet Nurse Smith*" instead of "Dr. Jones, this is Sally,* your nurse."

In the meantime, though, you are still probably not going to see last names on our badges. If you want to write us up, as I am sure this patient would have liked, we will be happy to spell our first names. We will also give you the last initial.

~~~

RN: "Ma'am if you're going to hide your crack pipe in your socks, please have the decency to advise staff who are undressing you that there is a sharp object. We don't want to get cut, much less write up a report that we were sliced by a crack pipe."

Patient: "Yeah, you right, I'm sorry. I was afraid if you found my crackers you'd take my shit."

RN: "Ma'am, I'm not interested in taking your snacks, just in getting you undressed without getting hurt myself."

Note: "crackers" and "shit" both refer to crack cocaine. The patient had her drugs in one sock and the crack pipe in the other.

~~~

MD to a patient in thick Asian accent: "Your knees are *crying* because you too fat, they can't hold you up; you go home lose weight, and your knees won't hurt anymore." (Same Detroit-born doc and the same result.)

~~~

MD: to a gay male patient complaining of painful hemorrhoids, a comment that would haunt this doctor for years as everyone who knows him or has ever heard of him will utter these five words with the same Asian accent: "Butt hole not for sex." I swear, go to Detroit, stand in the middle of any street, and utter those words. Someone will ask how in the world you know Dr. Ma.

~~~

RN: A 120 Kg patient (265 pounds), frustrated with waiting for a doctor, lowered herself to the floor to make an impact statement about her urgent need to see a physician. When told that the doctor was with a more critical patient, the patient insisted the nurse lift the patient back onto the gurney. The nurse responded, "What do I look like, Superman?"

~~~

RN: In the resuscitation module of a major city hospital, behind the curtain in Bay #1, a nurse instructed a medical student to do it, "Faster! Harder!" Unlike most TV and movie portrayals of hospital shenanigans, the nurse was simply instructing the medical student in how to do proper compressions (CPR) on a patient. Still...

~~~

Patient: A patient was trying to describe to a relatively new resident an implement she had used at home to expand her lungs after surgery. The resident did not understand that the patient was searching unsuccessfully for the words Incentive Spirometer, into which the patient blows against resistance to strengthen the lungs and help to prevent pneumonia. Exasperated, the delightfully genteel elderly woman looked at the doctor, and made one final attempt at description, "You know... the blow-jobby thing!"

~~~

MD: One ER resident did most of his assessment and orders from a desk. He hollered out questions to patients from across the room, extending the same lack of professionalism and courtesy to the ER staff expected to carry out his orders. The *curtain is not a wall* situation allows patients to hear what the medical staff declares as easily as those outside the curtain grasp what happens within the curtained patient care area.

A certain doctor habitually put his foot in his mouth as he yelled orders to secretaries and nursing staff. One secretary, Serina, tells me she was to order tests on the swollen lower legs of a morbidly obese patient who feared she had "blood clogs." The doctor hollered to Serina, for all to hear, "Can you get me Doppler's on those tree trunks in bed five?"

~~~

MD: The pharmacy called an ER nurse for clarification on an order that the physician had written, regarding the dosages of a rather large order of medications for a patient. The pharmacist wanted to know if the nurse was sure about giving those dosages, and if all of those medications were for the same patient. The nurse, sitting next to the doctor who had ordered the meds, relayed the questions, and the pharmacist clearly heard the answer directly from the physician. "Are you kidding me? She is a big fat pig.... Of course she needs all those meds, and she needs them in massive quantities." Yes, the same doctor who ordered Dopplers on the "tree trunks."

~~~

MD: "Discharge that patient in bed seven. She's not sick; she's crazy."

~~~

Patient: (who was about to get a pre-operative rectal exam from a 6'6" MD looked pleadingly at the doctor) "Can you please find me someone with smaller fingers? And preferably someone I don't know?"

The patient, an RN in that same facility, looked ever so relieved when the doctor, a colleague of many years, arranged for a medical student, an Asian female with tiny hands, to perform the examination.

~~~

MD: All of the doctors in a certain inner city ER carried phones with them so that staff could reach them at all times. Sometimes the doctors answered from the bathroom, made obvious by the sound echoing across the tiled enclosure. Instead of asking if it was an emergency or if the call could wait, the physicians occasionally shared too much information.

One doctor was particularly paranoid about germs, so his bathroom visits were long and involved. He took two towels, a washcloth, a bottle of alcohol, Tucks, and a magazine. The doc sanitized the bathroom and placed towels on the toilet seat to protect himself from whatever might live there. His paranoia was understandable, as certain cultures would not sit on the seat, often soiling it themselves while avoiding direct contact.

The doctor attempted his daily constitutional. During one of those in-bathroom phone calls, the doctor told the secretary requesting order clarification, "Serina, I'm pooping. I can't give you orders right now." Serina, revolted, did not call that doctor again for quite a while. Aversion therapy employed, score: Doc 1, Secretary 0.

~~~

RN: "Can I get some help over here? NOW?"

Those are the words that cause whoever does not have both hands busy to rush to the source of the request. A very confused elderly man with Alzheimer's did not take kindly to being away from home as dusk shimmied into darkness and he became more confused. We call it *Sundowners Syndrome,* or *Sundowning,* a medical mystery that may be from all of the accumulated stressors in the day overwhelming the patient, nighttime hormonal imbalances, or even simple fatigue.

Standing at 6'4" the patient was not at all a slight man, and the RN soon found that he packed a good wallop. He landed two right crosses before she could move out of his reach. With calming medications on board, a very sweet security officer, who had dealt with PTSD veterans, stayed and stroked the man's hand, speaking softly to him until the medications took effect.

~~~

ERT: (ER Technician) "Oh, no, you will NOT punch my nurse. You will NOT hit any staff member in this facility. Do you understand me?"

Hitting by a confused old man is forgivable. They do not know what they are doing. This time, it was a completely lucid middle-aged man.

The patient decided on this visit that he did not like the nurse starting the IV in his foot, the same place that the same nurse had done many times before. This guy was homeless with a history of seizures, did not like to take his meds, and came into the ER regularly for an IV boost of anti-seizure medications. As a bonus, he received a place to sleep, fresh clothing, and three meals a day (three hots and a cot).

Very often, the doctors would write an order to wash this patient's feet. He suffered from *toxic-sock syndrome,* an unearthly smell emitted by unwashed feet that live in the same pair of shoes 24/7. The procedure involved soaking the feet in shaving cream and then wrapping them in towels and plastic to kill the smell and loosen the debris.

The nurse, head down and concentrating on getting blood drawn and starting an IV in one of those lovely feet, did not see the swing coming. Fortunately, the tech, who was a staff sergeant in the US Army and recently returned from Iraq, did. The tech caught the swing and subdued the patient as gently as one could under the circumstances. Thank God for our soldiers, even in-country, for keeping us safe from harm.

~~~

Patient: "Do you think I could have another of those refreshing complimentary lemon custards? That was really good."

ER Staff: "Ma'am, we don't have any lemon custards."

Patient: "Sure you do... I found it in the bedside drawer."

The patient, an elderly female, had eaten the lemon-scented soft-gel room deodorizer from the bedside supply drawers. Since she was not the first to do this, we could no longer carry the lemony treats, much to the staff's chagrin. The lemon air fresheners were the most effective at warding off the unwanted scents of bodily fluids and toxic-sock syndrome not meant for polite company.

~~~

Patient: (when handed a KY Jelly packet from the bedside drawer to wet his dry lips, since he was not allowed to eat or drink anything), "Well, this is better than the Vagisil I brushed my teeth with the other day."

~~~

RN: Overhead between two staff nurses (30ish male to 50ish female): "You know you are kind of sexy... in a menopausal sort of way."

Thanks, Peter. You have such a great ... um... bedside manner.

~~~

RN: (Peggy, on the day of a full moon) "You know what we need? Valium aromatherapy, and a Vicodin salt lick for employees."

~~~

Patient: (laughing, when asked about her pain status after receiving narcotics for abdominal pain) "My belly feels fine, but my ass is asleep."

~~~

RN: (to another RN after standing over a patient they had been coding—CPR and resuscitative efforts—for 40 minutes) "my bladder is about to burst, and God help me if I get another patient right now. If it is anything short of death, I'll kill them myself."

~~~

MD: (at the end of a long and demanding day, humorously contemplating which option would be the greatest at stress relief) "I think I just want to sit in a hotel room and watch dirty movies."

~~~

RN: (Overheard by Tomi, exasperated by yet another patient with high dose pain meds for no discernible disease or injury, while sitting at the front desk charting her nursing notes.) "These people are F—n killing me with their 400mg a day OxyContin dosages."

A Schedule II controlled substance with an abuse liability similar to Morphine, docs prescribe OxyContin for Opioid-tolerant patients. These patients have been on pain medications for an extended period, and no longer get any relief from dosages less than 80mg every 12 hours. In some states, narcotics flow like water, so the potential for abuse is great. The street value is high if patients choose to sell their medications illegally. A single 40mg pill might go for $40.

~~~

Patient: The young female patient instructed the ER nurse as to what medications she wanted, how fast to push her 4 mg of IV Dilaudid, what tests she would allow, where to place the IV, and when she wanted all results and diagnoses. She had a hair appointment that afternoon. She also dictated what meal she wanted while waiting, and which doctor she preferred. When the RN tried to explain the hospital policy, procedures, and realistic time expectations to the patient, the patient said, "You are here to serve me." The nurse replied, "No ma'am that would be the Burger King down the street."

~~~

RN: Sue is from Toronto, which she claims is the most multicultural city in the world with many Asian inhabitants. Unlike the HIPAA-conscious society of the United States, first and last names appear on the unit whiteboard to identify which patient is in which area. In the case of a certain male patient, the board remained blank. His name? "Fuc Yu."

~~~

RN: "Sir, keep your arm straight. Keep your arm straight or the IV fluid will not go in. Sir. Sir the medicine is not going to go in if you bend your arm. Sir, please keep your arm straight."

The patient was a male in his forties, hit by a car while walking down the street at night. The car was traveling about 45 miles per hour, and the man's legs sustained fractures below the knees. The blood that was pooling on the floor at the end of the patient's gurney from the open fractures was interesting. There was a funny-colored liquid sitting on top of the blood, almost like a puddle of gasoline on wet pavement.

The man did not survive his injuries. In the match of pedestrian vs. automobile, the auto usually wins. It later saddened the nurse to realize she had missed an opportunity. She was not sure what she could have or should have said, but she became mindful of the fact that the last words the man would hear before he succumbed to his injuries and died, were, "Sir, please keep your arm straight."

~~~

Patient: (48-year-old female who had obviously had a facelift, chin and cheek implants, breast augmentation, nose job and way too many injections in her misshapen and disproportionate lips) "What is the point of being healthy if you don't look good?" Rumor has it, although I cannot verify, that she was also in the market to find a new plastic surgeon.

~~~

RN: A 35-year-old male patient came in with an amputated finger secured in a baggie filled with ice water, which the patient handed to the nurse. The nurse held onto the body part at the bedside, and when the doctor came to evaluate the wound, the nurse said, "I have always wanted to do this," and gave that doctor the finger.

~~~

Sometimes relaying exactly what happens in the nurse's notes can be entertaining when read by the oncoming shift. We crack up as we are writing it, knowing that the quotation marks, reflecting what the patient/doctor, etc. said, allow for entries one might not otherwise find socially acceptable. Some entries received judicious editing here out of respect for the varied reading audiences. Fill in the blanks.

Nurse's Notes

1530: "Patient not in assigned area, gown on bed, patient not found in hallway, waiting room, or smoking area. Doctor advised of situation, security and triage staff advised to watch for patient. Attempts by ER staff to call patient at home continue."

1605: "Patient called 911 from the main lobby of the ER, and made a bomb threat for this hospital after going to the hospital lunchroom and helping herself to food without paying. Food services staff called Security, patient escorted out of the cafeteria. Patient returned to the ER waiting room and made the phone call from an in-house phone. Security escorted patient back to bed in ER. Patient placed near nurse's desk, clothing and belongings removed, sitter at bedside, Doctor at bedside to re-evaluate, Psych evaluation ordered." Sometimes people just are not happy with the service no matter what you do.

~~~

1215: "Patient arrives via EMS with complaint of medication over-dose and syncope (fainting). Paramedics report that patient was up for two nights drinking, no sleep, no food, followed by ingestion of Ecstasy and other unknown recreational drugs. Patient drowsy but knows name, date, and place. Vital signs stable, monitor on, IV established, MD at bedside."

Further examination of the belongings, and questioning the patient, who appeared to be 16, revealed an ID for an Asian woman (the girl looked Latino) named Kenya*, age 33, another ID for Destiny,* and the girl admitted that her *professional* name was DeeLightFul.*

Her clothing included boots with 6" clear spiked heels, a mini-skirt, sequin-studded bra, G-string, see-through black halter top, and several additional pairs of panties that one surely wouldn't find at Wal-Mart. Dee* (DeeLightFul was a little clumsy, and Dee seemed more fitting for a teenager) finally admitted to being an 'exotic dancer' with no perm-anent address. Not what any mom might imagine for her teenage daughter.

We all shook our heads and then privately called our children, especially our daughters, to make sure they had everything they needed. I called mine and told her to fill her gas tank and get some groceries on my credit card. I told her to buy anything else she might need, understanding that she was on a limited budget, and I did not want to imagine her being hungry, cold, or in need. My daughter would pick up more shifts at the hospital if she needed money, of course, as she was responsible and independent. As parents, sometimes we help a little when our children have grown and gone, even if only to make ourselves feel better.

~~~

2230: "Pt arrives at ED #4 with a vague complaint of pain to abdomen, will not allow RN to assess, and says he will only speak with doctor. Girlfriend at bedside with patient, resident notified of situation."

2245: "ER Resident to bedside to examine patient, informs RN caring for patient that patient and his girlfriend were 'playing,' patient got a vibrator stuck in his rectum; awaiting x-ray, patient in no distress."

2315: "Resident to bedside to attempt to remove foreign object from rectum; unsuccessful. Second resident to bedside to make same attempt, unsuccessful. Surgery paged. Patient in no distress, medication (Valium 10 mg PO) given as ordered."

0100: "Surgical resident to bedside to remove foreign object from patient's rectum. Object successfully removed from patient and placed in sink. Object cylindrical in shape and vibrating loudly. Resident asked to disengage power supply to object as the noise is bothering nearby patients. Resident refused, gave verbal order to RN to disengage power."

~~~

1545: "Pulled a female out of a car, unconscious, shallow breathing, rapid pulse, pale, diaphoretic, clothing soaked with water. Female who dropped patient off states patient is a 15-year-old who was at a party, and may have taken some kind of drug, although the adult female who dropped patient off denies any drugs being on the premises."

Before the adult female had the chance to leave, (drop and run is common with a drug overdose, gunshot wound, not breathing, or in need of CPR), security escorted her back inside. She nervously anticipated talking to the police, who would have detailed questions. In the streets, the remedy for drug overdoses is dousing the person in ice water, and dropping them at the door of the nearest ER.

Security detained this *innocent until proven guilty* witness until the police arrived. As it turns out, the patient was an overachieving, scholarly, athlete who was supposed to be studying with a group of girls, and with parental permission. This young lady had never taken someone else's drugs before, and it almost cost her life. One time. One experiment.

When her very concerned parents were finally located and brought to the ER, they were stunned. "I never thought my daughter would do anything like this. She is the last person we would expect to be involved in this type of activity. We didn't even know she knew anyone who could get drugs, let alone take them herself."

Moral of the story? Parents who say, "My kid would never…" need to realize that their kid might. Keep a close eye and be there in case the unthinkable happens, because it does. It could happen to your kid.

~~~

1905: "Turned patient over to EMTP Sherry with full report and transfer paperwork. Patient's parents with him, medic carried patient to ambulance for transport to burn center. Patient in stable condition, IV of 0.9 NS running per burette, cool, moist compresses to burns on face, neck, chest, and back. Per MD at Children's Hospital, no medications are to be given for transport."

This is where the story usually ends for the ER nurse. She has completed care of her patient, called report to the receiving facility, and turned her patient over to EMS. For the medic who assumes care of the patient, it is another story as their work is just beginning. For this patient, a 10-month-old, with second-degree burns acquired by pulling a cup of scalding coffee over himself (that mom/dad left on the counter), it was the first step in a long process of treatment and recovery.

The other medic on the ambulance that day was Wayne, a single and egomaniacal, self-appointed super-medic, who had refined sexual harassment to an art. As a parent, and with some level of empathy still intact, I chose to attend (take care of the patient in the back of the ambulance). Wayne was out of the picture and into the driver's seat.

During that short walk from the ER to the ambulance, I had to deal with two arguing parents, whose voices increased in volume to drown out the other. They blamed each other for the child's injuries, for the potential keloid scarring to which people of color are prone. Those keloids, rubbery, painful, itchy, overgrowths of tissue, can affect skin movement.

The child was crying inconsolably, and the parents were concerned with their drama. Normally, family members do not ride in the patient compartment of an ambulance, but an exception can occur with children. The usual and expected response from the child is comfort when parents are nearby. In these instances, parents become my patients, too. My care extends to include them.

In this case, and at my request, the parents stopped their mutual attacks long enough to step inside the rig with their child and me. Mom did what she could to assist by hanging the IV bag on an overhead hook, and held the oxygen toward her son's face for blow-by administration. Dad's continuation of self-serving declamation pointed to a fork in the road, where empathy jumped out of the back of the truck and took a hike.

We should be empathetic and remember that the secondary patient, the parent, has needs, too. We are supposed to identify what is going on with this additional client, a dad whose son encountered a possibly disfiguring injury, and set value judgments aside. The dad in this situation was responding to his needs and experiences, and while he was not a priority at that precise moment, as a medic/RN, I always need to remind myself that brief reasoning might be helpful.

I told the dad that he had every right to be upset over his child's injury, but the long-term effects could not yet be determined, and the priority was taking care of the baby. One sentence of validation seemed to calm this father. Even though he was stuck in his response, and our goals were poles apart, that moment of substantiation seemed to help.

The father stepped out of the ambulance and drove his private vehicle behind us to the receiving facility. I continued to pour sterile saline over the boy's wounds to soothe them, soaking my uniform. The cooling fluids and some soft humming into the boy's ear, while rocking him back and forth in my arms, finally helped to calm him.

When we arrived at the burn unit, and I gave report to the receiving facility, we faced another confrontation. The father, still upset, was asked by the hospital personnel to "leave the facility until (he) could get it together." It seems the ride over gave Dad time to get angry again, and he immediately took it out on the receiving facility staff. They had even less patience than I did.

These types of calls happen every day for EMS and ER staff. It seems easy to step back, call the father a jerk, and detail how we would have handled that type of situation if our child sustained similar injuries. But do we know?

Looking back, I can honestly say I have never been a black male with all the associated cultural, social, and historical influences of that man. I do not know what his experiences were, or how important facial/bodily scarring might be for acceptance, ridicule, socialization, gaining employment in the future, etc. I have never experienced that man's struggles or teachings.

I do not know if he had knowledge of kindness, acceptance, or love. I do not know if he had the mental, physical, or spiritual tools to deal with adversity. I do not know of his belief systems or his sense of self-worth.

As a medical professional, I am to avoid having expectations of individuals, to recognize their inherent value, and *not to judge*. Behaviors do not define a person. They represent a thought process.

Putting ourselves in the client's shoes to identify with them and their feelings seems logical. It would allow a greater sense of empathy. However, if we get too close to the situation, if we identify with the pain and loss of the patient or his families, we can lose our objectivity and the ability to do our jobs well. We walk a fine line, a tightrope high above the ground, and we have no net.

~~~

0900: "Patient complains of (c/o) brain contracting. 'It feels like a laser in my brain,' Patient also c/o massive pain in the top left side of her head when the parasites bore in, very sudden bloody diarrhea, extreme fatigue, left eye soreness, slurred speech, vision problems, massive pain in left abdomen, trouble sleeping, severe anxiety, feeling as though she will 'black out or vomit when the parasites start biting and migrating in the abdomen,' pain to both legs and areas in chest, loss of appetite, bloating, nosebleeds, soreness in tailbone and right foot, itchy feeling at night around 'rear end,' sometimes loss of control of facial movements when parasites move around into certain areas of the brain, and 'hand tremors with bloody fluid from the vagina.'"

My sympathies go to the nurse, doctor, and social worker. I swear we do not make this stuff up.

~~~

0045: Pt states, "You already know my deepest secret. That I toyed with madness and lost."

Sometimes the things people say are heart wrenching because you can feel their pain and are helpless to do anything at that moment short of giving them some medication. An anxiolytic decreases anxiety and calms them. An anti-psychotic makes them manageable. Some complaints have no cure, just a stabilizing treatment so folks can function.

Some of their sharing includes, "You've never walked on the other side of the door (mental hospital), or been one to watch the holder of the key" (staff locking you in). Are these always street people who are drug and alcohol abusers? Not necessarily. They are sometimes professionals. They are the folks who work with you and me, who we do business with every day, but we do not know their deepest secrets.

So be kind. There is a fine line between them and us. Any one of us could cross it, or quite possibly already have.

~~~

It does not take much to make us happy. The things people take for granted-- sitting for five minutes during a 12 hours shift, eating, drinking, emptying one's bladder, a "break" (some folks DO get them)—are precious. Some other things, the benefits of the job, are downright luscious.

They help to make sense of a crazed and oft-misunderstood world that we love. We are admittedly trauma junkies. We adore working in a forgiving uniform that some have described as pajamas (scrubs) and tennis shoes that hide orthopedic inserts.

A Few of My Favorite Things

Top 10 Favorite things for ER staff members:

1. **Anything free, especially pens.** Drug reps gave nurses the plastic ones, saving the metal pens for the docs. Our position was that because we were the ones telling the residents what medicines to order, give *them* the cheap plastic pens. Pharmaceutical companies stopped giving incentives, as though they would influence someone's prescribing or practice, but we miss them.

2. **Pizza.** Even after a trauma. Quick, God's most perfect food, and no silverware required.

3. **Chocolate.** Better when individually wrapped, so we can put it in our pockets to nibble on between patients.

4. **Leftovers.** Even my mother learned years ago that if you have *any* food left over, bring it to the ER because it will be better than whatever the cafeteria fries up. The caveat is that we have to know you. In this society, people sabotage food, or might not be as clean as germaphobic ER folks would like.

5. **Anything you can safely wrap** in a paper towel and hide from predators for later ... assuming no one steals it.

6. **Coffee.** Lots of coffee, preferably NOT brewed on the premises. Tim Horton's or Dunkin Donuts will make me swoon. Most coffee makers in ERs have been there for several years, never cleaned, and probably dangerous. Do not drink from them unless desperate.

7. **Caffeine**. Failing coffee, we love anything containing caffeine. Warm pop/soda is better than tap water, as it usually contains the kick we need to get through the shift.

8. **Snack machine foods**. Peanut M&Ms, satisfying number three above with a little protein to assuage the guilt from eating chocolate, is portable and justifiable. One has to keep up one's strength, after all.

9. **Power bars**. High protein is best, and some are low-carb. They often taste like cardboard, but Mama always said if you get hungry enough, you will eat anything. She was right.

10. **Prescriptions**. Staff docs write tons of scripts for staff and EMS crews, avoiding a trip to the family doctor, waiting room time, and co-pay. Our docs will write what you ask for as long as you can justify the request. Of course, you usually ask for a remedy to fix something you caught in the ER, like upper respiratory stuff, or the urinary tract infection you got because you could not empty your bladder in a 12-hour shift.

~~~

Favorite discharge instructions for nurses to deliver to patients: "Stop doing drugs or you will die. Sign here, please."

~~~

Favorite three words for nurses to utter to Security Officers (armed agents with arresting authority): "Take Him Down." This means that the combative patient who tried to attack the nurse will have hands laid upon him by large men with handcuffs and guns who do not mess around.

The Security Officers will then put leather restraints on the patient securing him to the stretcher. The highly skilled ER techs will cut off the patient's clothing, holding the patient down at all bendable places. The nurse will administer a B-52, which is an intramuscular injection of Haldol 5mg and Ativan 2mg (hence the 52). The desired effect is to sedate the patient as quickly and safely as possible, so B for Bomber.

Following those actions, a very large bore needle (two are preferred) will be inserted for the administration of IV fluids and medications. Of course, there is a lifesaving Foley catheter, lest the unconscious patient urinates on himself, his bed, and anyone else within spraying distance. You know when that patient is regaining consciousness, because they will ask, often less than delicately, who put that tube in their … um… penis. We encourage them not to pull it out lest they become impotent for life.

~~~

Favorite form of entertainment and most important thing to teach new residents and worthy medical students: water fights. Mock H_2O (water) combat is a tradition in ERs, especially during the summer, and usually on the midnight shift. The shirts and skirts (management), ever present during the day, have no sense of humor, and do not see this activity as professional or safe. Harrumph.

If you fill a 20cc syringe with water and put a 22g catheter on the end of it, you can get tremendous distance. I love to tell a patient to, "Watch this," as I soak a resident across the room, and then turn my back. The patient gets to report the reaction, and the resident usually has no idea where the water came from, often looking at the ceiling for leaking pipes.

The 20cc syringe and 22g catheter give you great power, and the recipient of your playfulness never sees it coming. It is a skill and a joy to behold but try not to aim for the groin lest the recipient of the water look like they have just peed themselves. That is just wrong.

~~~

Favorite Attitude: Doctors with a sense of humor. The day goes by a lot better when your physician is as irreverent as you are. We want them to be medically proficient and get the job done, but in those moments between patients, we need to laugh. A doc with a sense of humor reduces our stress levels immensely.

One of those docs is DB. His initials also stand for "Dead Body," which is largely humorous on its own. Dr. Don B., who led our trauma center's residency program, recently retired from that responsibility after a lifetime of nurturing new kids right out of medical school. Don (we are on a first name basis with the best and most secure docs) loved to shock people and get a reaction from them, making work more like play in a place we called "Hell."

One day, while giving a female medical student (and potential resident) a tour of the ER, Don brought her through all of the seven modules (75 beds). As he traversed through the 11-bed module I worked that day, he stopped briefly at the nurses' station where I stood charting and pointed to his cheek. Knowing Don for many years, I saw that he wanted to show this potential employee that we were one big family, so I reached up to kiss him on the cheek.

When Don turned his head and kissed me dead on the lips, I grabbed an alcohol prep pad and scrubbed my lips while saying, "Ew, Ew, Ew, Ew, EW!" The female medical student stopped dead in her tracks with her mouth hanging wide open. Don laughed, the medical student probably visualized major sexual harassment lawsuits, and I got back to my charting. Funny thing; that student never made it into the residency program at our facility.

~~~

Favorite partner: one who doesn't smoke, has a large bladder, can talk and work at the same time, does not disappear from the work area, can keep up with his/her patients, and at some point during the shift asks if you need any help. S/he is your best friend for all 12.5 hours of your shift, never touches your IV tray to steal supplies and covers your patients during lunch. It does not get much better than that.

~~~

Favorite uniform: Admittedly, getting a job that allows you to wear clothing that is cotton, shape-conforming, figure-forgiving, has an elastic or tie waist, and goes with tennis shoes is not all bad. God bless whoever designed scrubs. The required color in our ER was navy-blue, which I have worn my entire nursing career. Dark colors hide bodily fluids, like charcoal (taken orally by overdose patients, often sprayed and splashed up to10 feet from the cup in which it is delivered), and iodine, which looks a lot like blood to the untrained eye.

~~~

Favorite task: Starting IVs. After multiple failed eye surgeries, and unsuccessful attempts to repair the botched PRKs (Photorefractive Keratectomy), I began to mourn the loss of my favorite skill. It became a point of interest to see how long I could go with the visual impairment before finding a patient upon whom I could not successfully, regardless of numbers of attempts, gain Intravenous (IV) access. It never happened.

The most hilarious patients are those who have a history of IVDA (IV Drug Abuse), who have used up their veins and are deficient in anything ER-poke worthy. They will point to the one or two they still use, but those bits of veins cannot support IV catheters. Many patients requested me by name to start their IVs, and other nurses would poke multiple times before accepting defeat and coming to get me. Unfortunately, I would establish a saline lock only to find that the patient, grateful for a way to get a reusable access for their drug habits, would walk out the door. I often wonder if they bragged about their semi-permanent line for street drugs, provided free of charge by the local trauma center.

~~~

Favorite ER complaint of all time: It still makes me shake my head. Unlike the lint in the belly button or hangnail complaints, which happened, this one would be *so* embarrassing. I do not know how a patient would consider this an ER-worthy visit. Especially *twice.*

A teenaged female was in a car moaning and thrashing about while her mother came running to the security gate. Mom, panicking, told the officers she needed a gurney right away for her daughter, who was in too much pain to get into a wheelchair. The Security Officers called triage yelling for a gurney. The triage nurse dropped everything and went outside to get the girl, fearing critical gunshot or stab wounds.

What she found was a morbidly obese teenage female who was complaining of rectal pain. The girl was wearing a thong not designed for her girth, causing irritation to her rectum. She was discharged an hour later in a wheelchair.

The next day the same nurse was working at the triage desk when that same mother came running into the Security Officers. Mom said she needed a gurney for her daughter, who was in too much pain to get into a wheelchair or walk into the ER. The nurse stopped staff from running out with a stretcher and told the mom to walk or wheel her daughter into the ER. There would be no more driveway rescues for impacted thongs.

~~~

Favorites from outside the double doors: Cops and Medics. Once a medic, always a medic; the yen for working the road never leaves you. However, somewhere along the way I got too old to scrape folks off the street at 3 a.m. in the dead of Midwestern winters, so my brothers in blue, whether EMS or Police, are always a welcome sight. I adore them, I envy them, I cherish them, and I cannot imagine the world without them.

Jeff Bare is a former PA Chiefs of Police Project and CISM Team Coordinator whom I have adopted as a brother. He keeps me sane. Jeff puts it into a nutshell: "Police are the only warriors on the battlefield who run toward the sounds of the guns, the others run to retreat. They are the only ones who can save a life, take a life, or bring a life into the world."

From the Medic side, there are always stories, especially from Rob. The last pearl Rob gave me was about a student of his (EMT class) who went to the front of the class to practice a trauma assessment. The student started out strong, finding all the imaginary injuries. He suddenly became quite nervous, losing his focus, and stating that the right-sided injuries were on the left. Rob watched the student's anxiety increase as he approached the abdomen for assessment. When it came time to *verbalize* the genitalia exam, the student said, "I now *oralize* the genitalia." He sat down after the laughter subsided, and dropped the class a week later.

~~~

Sometimes people ask how we in EMS/ER handle our jobs, especially in life and death situations. The truth is, sometimes stress is not stressful, especially when we get to do the impossible and make a difference. We find the experiences exhilarating and addictive; they feed us.

This story is about doing the impossible. A high-five moment, it left us pumped-up and ready to face the next challenge. These situations keep us going after too many days of inane drama and "you can't fix stupid."

I'm NOT Letting You Go

I held a woman's life in my hands today. It may sound a bit melodramatic, but as I watched the blood spurting from her neck and saw her gaze fearfully into my eyes, the reality of what we do in an Emergency Center hit hard. As staff nurses in a 75-bed trauma center, we deal with life and death every day. Occasionally we covertly and carefully slip out of clinical mode to realize the fragility of human life and address our mortality. This was one of those moments.

Cynthia* presented as a 42-year-old woman with a recent history of tongue, larynx, and voice box removal secondary to cancer. The procedure was one month old, and she bore the physical evidence of surgery with drains and healing suture lines on her left carotid (neck) area. She had been coughing up blood since that morning and came to us via ambulance at 0900. We assessed her airway, determined it to be patent (open), and Sandy (the respiratory tech) prepared the tracheostomy mask. Dr. Marson*, anticipating changing the tracheostomy tube, stepped away for just a moment while Sandy attached the humidified oxygen.

"I need a doctor here, NOW!" Sandy called from the bedside. She was behind curtain six in an 11-bed module, and the nursing station was just a few feet away. The patient was partially out of view of the nurses, and this was an emergent situation.

Sandy put a gloved hand over Cynthia's spurting carotid artery on the side of her neck and called for 4X4's (gauze). We gloved up, donning masks and goggles in the seconds it took to reach Sandy and Cynthia. Dr. Marson was already there and continued applying pressure to the site.

We rechecked Cynthia's vitals and found that her SpO2 (oxygenation) had dropped to 90% on the mask (it was 99% before). Her blood pressure was reading relatively low at 86/42, and her heart rate shot up to an unacceptable tachycardic rate of 132. In a matter of seconds, Cynthia pumped out at least 200 ccs of blood through her left carotid artery. We suctioned another 200 ccs from her tracheostomy and oral cavity.

We called for additional staff to our area. Cynthia was too unstable to move to the resuscitation module where there was more room and better equipment, and we began the process of stabilizing her. The doctor established a central line; we sent lab samples for a type and screen, called for two units of blood, and hooked warmed saline to Cynthia's triple lumen IV catheter, running wide open. Cynthia's lungs were clear, so we hung a second IV fluid bolus of warmed saline and attempted to make her as comfortable as possible with warmed blankets while we continued to hold pressure to the site of her arterial bleeding.

After 10 minutes, with surgery paged and the vital signs returning to a more acceptable 102/58 and heart rate of 94, we slowed the fluids. We assessed Cynthia's lungs and airway and continued to reassure her. Cautiously, we administered 2mg of Morphine Sulfate slow IV push for the post-op pain from her left shoulder reconstructive surgery.

I assumed the position of holding pressure on the left carotid artery and stood over her for another 20 minutes while we awaited the surgeons' arrival. We monitored her airway and vital signs. I maintained eye contact and softly reassured her that we would take good care of her, and make her as comfortable as possible.

After a total of 30 minutes of direct arterial pressure, the bleeding stopped, airway secured, and vital signs stayed within normal limits. We stepped cautiously aside to permit surgeons to assess our patient. The plan was for Cynthia to go to the OR at a time yet to be determined.

We also cared for the other 10 patients in the module while keeping a watchful eye on this very critical young woman. The ENT (Ear Nose and Throat) resident had evaluated Cynthia and then left our module in an attempt to expedite the surgical team. Cynthia showed no further signs of bleeding, and we thought the immediate danger had passed, when suddenly a general surgery resident at the bedside called for help.

This inexperienced resident thought it would be a good idea to wiggle a line that was coming from the healing neck wound, which caused the blood to come pouring out again. This short and apparently intellectually challenged female resident was quickly moved aside, and despite her protestations and exclamations of, "But I'm a doctor," was relieved of duty by the patient's primary nurse. Fortunately, we did not see that resident again for the rest of the day. ER nurses can become Mama Bears when it comes to protecting our patients.

In those few seconds, my partner, Nurse Christine, watched about 300 ccs of blood saturate the 4X4s and pool under Cynthia's neck. We asked the secretary to contact the blood bank to send another four units of blood stat, called for more staff, again summoned the surgeons to check on the availability of an OR (we needed it NOW), and switched positions. I put pressure on Cynthia's neck as my partner suctioned her tracheostomy tube (not too deeply, as we did not want her to cough and force pressure on the carotid artery). Cynthia motioned for the Yankaur Suction set and suctioned her oral airway. That action permitted a small piece of control in a situation where she felt she had little to do with outcomes.

I explained to Cynthia what was going on, reassuring her while looking into her eyes that we were *not* going to give up. We would fight for her. We proved our tenacity by protecting her from a resident who lacked the critical thinking skills necessary to determine that one does not wiggle a line coming out of a bleeding carotid artery. That part was fun.

No blood was oozing out of the wound site as evidenced by the dry stack of 4X4s under my fingers. I braced myself for a long wait while staff prepped the OR. The vascular surgeon was making his way to our medical center from another location, expected arrival time indeterminate.

We gave Cynthia another 2mg of Morphine Sulfate IVP for pain, and to help relax her, added pressure bags to the infusing blood, and continued stabilization measures while the minutes ticked away. I applied pressure over the artery with my right hand and held Cynthia's left hand with my own. I looked into her eyes and made jokes about how we were awfully close to each other for having met just a few hours before.

She pulled my nametag down, looked at it, and attempted a smile. I said, "Yes, I'm Sherry. You'll remember that tomorrow when you wake up with a sore neck from my leaning on you." She nodded, knowing that I was silently praying for her as fervently as she was for herself.

Everyone calmly pitched in during Cynthia's care. An ERT, Bonnie, grabbed my waist-length hair out of a failing band and collected it from me in a braid to keep it from becoming contaminated in the blood. Our secretary, Renee, covered my feet in booties and placed a hair net over my newly fashioned braid. Another tech ran to get masks, gowns, and goggles for the gathering staff, placing them on each staff member at the bedside asking, "what else do you need, what can I do for you?"

No voices raised, everyone was calm, and the process was seamless. The patient representative, Dee, found Cynthia's family members to get the appropriate consents signed as another nurse placed a monitor on the stretcher. At about 100 pounds, Cynthia did not take up much space, so there was plenty of room for her, the monitor, and me sitting beside her, still holding pressure. My fingers were numb, cold, and cramping. My arm was shaking, but I was not going to let go. To release that artery was to let go of Cynthia's life, and I was not willing to take that risk.

I rode the cart upstairs and delivered Cynthia onto the OR table, trading places with a surgeon who assumed my position of holding pressure. I reported that Cynthia had received three and a half liters of saline, was completing her second unit of blood and four more units were on the way to the OR. Her vital signs were stable, and she was alert throughout the ordeal. She received a total of 4 mg of Morphine IVP and was relatively comfortable. We were amazed that she made it to the OR and wondered for the rest of the day about her outcome.

The ENT resident who had originally evaluated Cynthia came down to the Emergency Department later to thank us (yes, that is quite unusual), saying that he appreciated what we had done. He reported that those types of patients *do not make it* to the OR, so we had done some amazing work. The young doctor told us that surgeons ligated the artery, and they were watching Cynthia closely in SICU. They hoped against odds that she would survive without further complications, such as a stroke. Sandy (the respiratory tech) told me months later that Cynthia had survived the ordeal and was improving, still remembering the nurse who sat on the cart with her and would not let go.

Cynthia's face is still vivid in my mind. I held her life in my hands. It was a blessing, a privilege, and a responsibility I do not take lightly.

In medicine and nursing, we sometimes become a little too hardened. Our clinical trauma armor allows us to do our job effectively without overwhelming emotional attachment. However, this time, the connection strengthened my resolve that this patient would not die on my watch.

I held her life in my hands as God held my hand steadily over hers. These are the moments that reaffirm why we do what we do, and renew pride in our profession. We do the type of work that not everyone can do.

4	**Corrections** **Prison Health Care Stories** **from Nurses, COs, and Staff**

The intent of this section is to take a cross-eyed look at life within the corrections (jail, prison) system. During my first week of working in a high-security state facility, I saw several nurses and corrections officers roll their eyes at the drama of Women with a Penis, or as they called it, Mangina Syndrome. My funny bone reverberated like a tuning fork, and it felt fabulous. For those who do not speak medical, the definitions for Mangina and Angina are different despite sounding alike. Remember: tongue in cheek.

I felt like Alice stepping through the looking glass into a world I could never have imagined. Despite numerous television and movie efforts to educate about the other side of the clanging metal doors, you have no concept of their reality until you clear the gate. There is so much to tell, so few pages in which to tell it. What I share in this section reflects the thoughts, feelings, and experiences of various corrections personnel. Medics and RNs who deal with patients in the custody of Law Enforcement Officers (LEOs) also share a few thoughts.

You will read anonymous contributions from prison nurses, corrections officers (COs), medical, and mental health staff in and outside of the prison system. Much of the information contained in this section intends to give you an idea of our experiences, good or bad, and the reality of working in a place that society would prefer to ignore. We are at the bottom of the occupational hierarchy, so we devise ways to endure. Our first goal is getting home alive and unharmed at the end of the day, how we get to that point varies. What we all share is humor.

Gallows humor is part of the culture of emergency responders, especially applicable in the structured systems of dealing with persons awaiting trial, in police custody, or convicted inmates. Working in prison health care as an RN/QMHP (registered nurse/qualified mental health professional), and balancing full-time doctoral studies, reinforced my appreciation for humor. If you stop laughing, you start crying. So laugh (when and where appropriate). Gleefully, joyfully, with complete abandon, laugh. Find the underside of tense situations and reframe them with hope and humor. Kindly laugh at others but most importantly, remember to laugh fully at yourself.

As you prepare to read this next section, sit down with your favorite beverage and get comfortable. Spend time with me through the following pages exploring the other side of the cuffs. When we have good days, we find the silliness in life. The George Carlin, Robin Williams, Stephen Colbert moments that make you pause, think, chuckle inwardly, or fall headlong into a belly laugh. Anyone who is big on political correctness should flip to the next section or close their electronic reader because I do not promise PC (politically correct) sensitivity.

This is how *some police, firefighters, paramedics, EMTs, nurses, corrections officers, and public service folks think and feel about working with the incarcerated. The jobs are dangerous. We are aware, but focusing on the negatives would drain us, so we look for the positives and occasionally the opportunities to laugh.

For those who are young or riding the Gandhi/Mother Theresa train, blessings to you unto the third and fourth generation. I am as caring as the day is long, but if the emotional tank does not refuel, the vehicle sputters and dies. Laughter is how we refuel.

Man·gi·na [man-jahy-nuh] Syndrome

Noun, plural man·gi·nas

Derivative of *angina*, a medical condition related to the heart; see below

1. Derisive term for a mammal of either sex lacking the qualities of maturity, especially under circumstances involving threat to health, well-being, emotional or physical injury, illness, or medical procedures including the swift removal of Band-Aids

2. Slang for those lacking the machismo (*aka* cojones) normally attributed to the testosterone-enhanced male population, or particularly gutsy females

An·gi·na [an-jahy-nuh]

Noun

1.   Squeezing chest pain representative of heart disease

2.   Popular media representation: "This is The Big One, Elizabeth! I'm coming to join ya, honey!"

*Names changed to protect the anonymity of corrections workers around the country who choose to give voice to the coping mechanisms that get them through the day.

Prison: We Just Work There

I have always known that Plato's Cave was an image, and had to decide whether to find a way out or stay in its secure womb. Lessons are sometimes painful for those journeying out of intellectual and emotional darkness. Internal evolution requires intense effort.

Therefore, those who shroud themselves with caves of ignorance or live on the perimeters of darkness (thinking they are in light) warrant tolerance, as it is their truth. Sometimes the difference between them and us, the inmate and the staff member, is almost indistinguishable. Sometimes the separation consists only of a Sally Port and a buzzer.

Prison is a community, a subculture that calls anything outside its walls *The World*. Those concrete walls, Sally Ports, and layers of barbed wire confine a separate reality. You find people who live within a new social order, a culture that takes care of its own; that applies rough justice and penalties by its code of conduct. Mirroring how they survived in The World, inmates actions emerge from need, connection (like gangs), power, and circumstance.

The prison is the inmate's home. We who go back to houses in The World at the ends of our shifts need to realize that we just work at the prison. Inmates will tell you they are in charge.

The inmates are running the asylum, they say, and simply allow people wearing uniforms and badges to *think* they have control. A constant battle for power wages between staff and inmates, and though they may not win the war, inmates will push the envelope through small skirmishes. They will find or create a battle they can win.

Things as small as bottom bunk privileges, special shoes, or challenging the speed of medication dispensing become issues. They will attempt to split staff with praise or cutting remarks. "Nurse Jones, you are the best. Not like that Nurse Kristen, she mean to me. You always nice and you care about me."

If inmates can get an extra Band-Aid, a packet of Tylenol, or a no-charge visit in medical with the nurse, they feel empowered. The power struggle is relentless. Currency is more than dollars. The value of information about the staff traded between inmates is priceless, often used against staff in the court of prison justice. I am Nurse Jones because like in the ER, I do not want inmates to have my full name lest they feel the urge, as many promised, to look me up when released.

We who come in from The World recognize a need for something to help us deal with those who have made life decisions so starkly contrasting and disharmonious with our own. Listening to the stories of inmates is not always easy, as they justify why they took someone's life or find momentary relief from pain by cutting deep grooves into their flesh. When the conversations have no value, become personal or argumentative, we practice the advice of my greatest mentor. Randi, RN, suggested simply, "Do not engage the prisoner." Silence is sometimes more than golden.

One staff member gently describes the environment as "different." "From the crazy inmates to the promiscuous officers, not to mention the politics in the hierarchy of custody, you have to be on your game every minute inside the perimeter. I have seen things I cannot unsee."

"I have seen guys hanging from light fixtures, flinging feces out of their food slot, eating their feces, eating plastic bags, slashing open cheeks. *Snitches get stitches* is practiced here, so they have that scar to wear for the rest of their lives. They make shanks from plastic bags. They bite each other."

"I saw an inmate marry a former nurse in the waiting room. I know of officers marrying inmates after they parole. I see things smuggled in like heroin, cell phones, marijuana, and tattoo guns. How it happens is unclear, but it happens. All of this happens, and if it were to broadcast on television people would declare it unbelievable."

Respect is huge in the prison system. Many inmates will tell you they will not give it if they do not get it, and to disrespect a prisoner, in their eyes, deserves harsh punishment. You may give them a look, a misinterpreted word, or accidentally bump into them. Those who have life sentences may take pleasure in inflicting pain on others, including staff, as they do not have anything to lose. Placement into *The Hole* (segregation cells, solitary confinement) is just a different vantage point of another day in the same old place.

The prison is a building surrounded by layers of sharp, shiny, barbed wire. Determining the purpose of prisons depends on whom you ask. The inmates look at forced confinement and loss of freedoms as a punishment for crimes committed by, or the fault of, someone else.

Mass incarceration, though not perfect, is far better than previous practices of public torture and execution. Enlightenment comes slowly.

Prisons house convicted persons, prevent escape, allow controlled supervision, and provide somewhat humane living arrangements until release or parole. Maintaining the security and safety of everyone inside and outside the facility is the highest priority. Enforcement of that security can get ugly when attitudes surrounding the inmates or their crimes become an issue. Providing what some see as unearned *freebies* to inmates, especially law libraries, education, and health care, can become a cause of disagreement that affects some staffs' attitudes.

Bad attitudes are not prevalent but they do exist, and they may show up in duty performance. Some nurses may display negative *enthusiasm* while administering medical care, but people are people. Not everyone is nice. Not every nurse is nice. Not everyone received a Florence Nightingale pin upon graduation from nursing school. Some nurses should flip burgers.

Gang mentality translates to strength in numbers. When any situation devolves to *us against them*, for any reason, people on either side of the cuffs can practice poor behaviors, and display less than stellar attitudes. We hope that other nurses or officers will step in to redirect attitudes to a more professional position. Mistreating detained or imprisoned patients is cruel and bullying. I will not suffer bullying.

~~~

Corrections Nurses: PC is not Practiced Here

When I moved from ED trauma to an inpatient closed psych ward and then to prison nursing, I thought my trauma nursing skills would wither and die. In my interview for the corrections nurse position, the manager asked if I was not just a little overqualified. With a bachelor's degree in management, a master's degree in psychology and working on a doctorate in education, on paper it may have seemed like overkill.

In my mind, it was barely enough. I was interviewing to work in the section of the prison housing high-security inmates with the compounding factor of mental illness. I felt barely qualified and kept my degrees in a front pocket, calling on their teachings rather often to get through some sticky situations.

When asked in the interview why the manager should hire me, *because I am cute* fell out of my mouth without filtering through any brain cells. Humor, remember? We had to acclimate: me to prison, and prison to me.

Asked how she adjusted to working in a prison after coming from a neat, clean, organized, well-stocked hospital, Libby tells me she had to learn the culture. "It took time to get over calling your patients 'Hun' and being touchy-feely towards them. It was hard at first [in corrections] to hear coworkers cursing and being disrespectful not only to inmates but also to each other. This is not an exception, either; it is the norm. I have learned to give quality medical care while having appropriate correctional standards."

Nurses in corrections are at the bottom of the hierarchical structure. Many are at the beginning of their careers and could not find other jobs, or they are waiting out retirement and could not find other jobs. They can be painfully inexperienced or bitter desk jockeys.

Very few nurses in corrections feel valued. Unlike in The World, where officers extend appreciation and respect to trauma nurses, many corrections officers view nurses as a hindrance. Some officers, like a dog on a meaty bone, refuse to let go of a story about how one nurse (secretary/mental health professional/teacher) got involved with an un-named inmate years ago. Therefore, all female staff members think with their loins and not their brains. Sorry, we are just not that into incarcerated bad boys.

Nor are we that into COs. True, I know some very happily dating and married COs and nurses, and some work at the same facility. However, like female paramedics who are not eager to jump into the back of a rig with every male EMS partner, not every nurse comes to work searching out a hot (or not) CO. Questioning nurses' judgment and competency by discounting their professionalism does not help the working relationship. Moreover, we do not carry Tasers, which is probably a good thing, as we might not resist the temptation to dry stun some frisky COs.

To be fair, sometimes the negative competency view is justified, as the Clueless Carol* types with elevated self-images, and substandard clinical judgment, want to rush into a medical scene without any assurance of safety. Those nurses get hurt. Those nurses get other people hurt.

They tarnish the reputations of real nurses blessed with brains and experience. They are the nurse want-to-be types who put the "B" in bureaucracy (and the other "B" word), doing little to earn government-issued paychecks in jobs from which folks rarely if ever receive a *pink slip*. Some prison nurses personify the Peter Principle, rising to the levels of their incompetence.

The other nurses are amazing. Real nurses who care, sometimes a little too much, and provide a momentary haven where inmates may focus on medical needs and issues and not their crimes. Nurses do not enforce the law or pass judgment. Prison health care can and should be a place where nurses assess physical and emotional wounds without acrimony.

Nurses can provide a bridge of non-judgmental respect while aware of the dangers around them. Moreover, nurses are aware of cameras, too. Most of us appreciate knowing that Big Brother (Control) is watching.

Because of one staff member's lack of judgment (not a nurse), RNs were admonished not to dance on the job. Cameras are everywhere and caught someone twerking in front of inmates. Publicly shaking your bottom is not a good coping practice in a prison and not the place to shake what your mama gave you.

My methods of survival and regeneration involved finding the Pollyanna moments and gaining assurance that I was making a positive difference in a very dark place. Seeking the bright side of situations allowed me to practice therapeutic nursing without judgment or rancor. It became a mantra.

Telling nurses not to believe inmates, because they always lie, creates distance. It makes it harder for nurses, who try to provide that singular haven inside the walls without succumbing to manipulations. Critical thinking, awareness, observing body language, and reading between the lines means survival for those who have nothing more than a little garage-door-opener-looking box with a string attached to pull in an emergency (PPD: Personal Protection Device). Better to anticipate and overcome problems before they begin. If you have to pull that string, you hope it works, and everyone comes running.

~~~

Corrections Officers: Subculture within a Subculture

*Sgt. Sunshine is into her second decade working within the prison system. She tells me that the nickname reflects a sincere appreciation from fellow officers for her positive attitude and ability to cheer coworkers. Making "cynical, miserable people" look at things from another vantage point offsets what a few male COs saw as detrimental:

attractive female with a bubbling personality in law enforcement. However, people skills are invaluable. The ability to calm inmates in distress or neutralize escalating situations is priceless.

There are dark times, too. "A sergeant and a CO went into a female inmate's segregation cell and beat the shit out of her. They said she was always talking crap and causing trouble. They both got fired."

"Then there was the female who went out on a writ (court order) to the county. She was knocked-up (impregnated) by a male convict who was a porter. We had to keep strapping her to the bed because she kept trying to kill the baby."

Golf* tells me his family was quite surprised when he became a CO. His family had always seen him as a "laid back type of guy, not professional, by the book, firm, and aggressive [when necessary]. Working in corrections does something to a person. It made me slow down and realize the things I have, to be grateful for them.

"There was a time in many CO's lives where they can tell you that they were almost in that same position [as the inmates], which could have ended them up in trouble or prison. Working in a prison also makes me more aware of my surroundings, to treat everyone the same, but to remain guarded.

"I love my job. I look back at my years with Corrections and compare them to other's in the prison system, or back at the academy, and I thank God I wasn't put in a bad regime or bad conditions. That affects a person mentally and physically. I've seen people totally change into something you would never think they could become. It helped to shape me. I may not like the work at times, but hey, that's why we get a good salary."

Kenzie* tells me, "We work a job that everyone is afraid of, but The World never really talks about what we do. They just know it's a scary place and bad people go there. We are referred to as guards, but guards watch things like banks and jewelry stores. COs protect the public from harm, motivate/rehabilitate offenders, protect offenders from other inmates. We are not guards, but sometimes you just don't feel like explaining [what we do], or giving details about work."

COs are part of a subculture of law enforcement. They do not get the same respect as uniforms outside the gate. I asked an NYPD detective if LEOs outside the system had an opinion about LEOs in correctional facilities. His perspective, which he says reflects conversations he has had with fellow detectives, is candid, and not intended to offend, but to inform.

I asked the detective if he could shed any light on the difference between street cops and corrections officers. He said, "Integrity. I think when they start out they're not corrupt. However, some begin with a disillusioned idea of what their future is going to be.

"When they get to where they're going, they realize that they're spending the job locked up for 20 years, just like the inmates. Then they have this incredibly increased exposure to hardcore criminals. Some of the COs can get a chip on their shoulders because everybody talks about street cops but nobody wants to hear about the corrections officers' day. They can start to feel jaded and abused. They can feel the pinch of their salary because they don't have time to think about much else except their horrible situation and the temptation of graft."

Mack gives his perspective as a career CO degreed in criminal justice. "A good CO is a person who is dedicated to their work and works hard to provide a safe work environment for the staff and a safe living situation for the prisoners. At times, they go beyond their normal duties and are not recognized for the hard work they do on a daily basis.

"Street cops get all the recognition and dislike corrections officers period, which I think comes from a lack of understanding of what we do. It is totally stupid. COs have to be constantly on guard with even the smallest things that may slip by a civilian. Those things can mean life or death, so working corrections gets you some of the best training in life."

However, Mack does acknowledge that sometimes the job and situation may change people. "With that being said, COs can become a little institutionalized because of the environment they're in. The bad ones can become disillusioned and corrupted by negative actions from supervision, or problems with personal finances. Those are the main two reasons that I have seen causing officers to fall from grace."

Sgt. Golden Eye adds a military perspective to viewing corrections officers. Asked if there was a difference between military and civilian, he focused on the military's team attitude that transcends duty assignments. "In the military, you have more of a connection. You do more than just work together; you live together in the same barracks or on the same base. It is more of a bond than with civilian corrections officers.

"There is no real negative stigma between corrections and MPs (military police/*multi-purpose*). I was an MP and never went to CO school, but worked in corrections. Corrections departments are small in the military. Everyone knows everyone, and we were called cage-kickers, but that was all in fun."

I loved *most* of my COs. People are people; some are amazing and made me feel safe, others did not impress. Unfortunately, the one stray gives a bad name to the 100 good that went before him. Like the nurse who married an inmate and tarnished the reputations of nurses forever in some COs eyes, one bully in a uniform can tarnish the image of a corrections officer.

In training, we are all told not to reveal personal information to the prisoners. If inmates know something about you, they can use it against you. They can threaten your family.

If a CO does a kindness for an inmate, the fallout can be negative. Inmates trade information about staff like currency, trying to get an upper hand, a break, a bit of control over their world. I hate to think of COs or nurses succumbing to the temptation of breaking the law for an inmate, whether for profit or to protect their family, but it happens.

~~~

Health Care: A Day in the Life of Prison Nurses

Dealing with incarcerated patients presents challenges for nurses. Patients on their way to incarceration, or temporarily relieved from confinement with a medical pass, pose unique problems and perspectives. Nurses' duties include responding to emergencies in the housing units (where the inmates live and sleep), the yard (exercise areas, walkways), and other buildings, like the library and chow hall. The practice of getting to the health care building to start each shift becomes an adventure before the job begins. Walk with me ...

Employees park in a lot far from the main building. The daily procedure begins with stepping out of the vehicle after taking one long, last sip of coffee/pop as you cannot bring it into the building, and patting yourself down. Do you have your car keys? Where is your cell phone? Are pockets empty, and everything you carry into the building contained in a clear, plastic purse or box (of specific dimensions)?

Lock your car and peek inside, reassuring that nothing of value is visible. Put your cell phone in your trunk, and hide or disguise valuable trunk contents. I hide my purse in a ratty cardboard box under partially empty containers of gluten-free protein bars. Seeing the healthy and tasteless packages of food-mimicking snacks, any self-respecting thief would move along to pillage the next vehicle.

Pat yourself down again before stepping away from the car. Question whether you completed all required steps, and especially that your cell phone is not on your person. Bringing cell phones into the prison is cause for immediate dismissal. Part way to the door, walk back to your car one last time to confirm that you locked it. One becomes appropriately cautious, or paranoid, depending on your perspective.

During inclement weather, that first tenth of a mile is not fun. I am a Michigan-born can-handle-cold-weather person who avoids wearing a coat until there is no other choice. My cold-weather selection is a navy blue jacket, with *St. John Emergency* emblazoned across the back in bright white letters. The coat stands up to below zero temperatures and announces to all within 40 feet that I am indeed a badass trauma nurse from Detroit.

Inside the first building, we grab our keys (picture the key ring of a high-school janitor), punch in, and wait in line outside the gate. The gate is inside a Sally Port, with two large glass doors at each side, and a walk-through metal detector. As you wait in line, you pull off outer garments and check pockets for contraband.

All food and drink are contraband. Pat yourself down again, and wait. We may give ourselves away in public, and in civilian clothes, by doing a pat down. If I check for my pen, ID badge, or PPD in the middle of the grocery story, go ahead and laugh.

If Corrections Officers enter the line outside the gate, they step in front of you (hierarchy). If a line of prisoners comes to the gate with transport COs, you step aside. Allow 30 minutes to get from car to workstation.

When instructed to step through the gate, hand the CO your coat, so she can inspect the pockets. Lay pens, keys, and ID badge on the counter, and walk through the metal detector. Time and experience tell which items will pass through without setting off the alarm.

If your coat is fluffy enough and the gate CO friendly enough, you can sometimes smuggle a bagel or a power bar through by tucking them into the gloves in your pocket. The CO will look down and whisper, "Food?" You look up and say, "Yeah; I have an extra pair of gloves and hat." It becomes a game.

Confession: I walked into the gate after lunch one day with my cell phone in my shirt pocket. The gate alarmed and I immediately reached for my phone saying, "Oh, crap, I forgot ..." The gate CO, a female to whom I will be forever grateful, immediately slapped my breast pocket closed whispering, "There are cameras. You could be fired. Take that back to your car."

I did as she suggested, amazed that I could have made such a stupid mistake. We laughed about that day for a long time. The CO describes it as the unexpected benefit of being "felt up" by your gate CO.

Gather your belongings, sign in on the gate clipboard, accept your PPD from the CO inside another secured enclosure, and shove everything in your pockets before the second glass door opens. Knowing that you will probably not get a break or lunch, hitting the pop and snack machines for caffeine and sugar becomes a habit. When sufficiently assembled, you wave at the Control officers behind the glass indicating that you are ready for them to buzz you into the yard.

You walk another 105 steps to the front door of the medical building, acknowledging staff and inmates along the way. To ignore them is rude, and may indicate, to the inmates, a level of discomfort or fear. Inmates can smell fear.

You are appropriately friendly, polite, and respectful. If you have a good relationship with the inmates, one of them will race ahead of you to hold the door open. Respect and courtesy go a long way in this environment. So do attempts at manipulation, but either way, the door opens.

After acknowledging the CO assigned to your building, you briefly exchange pleasantries and sign in to your work building. Peeking into each exam room, you let staff know you have arrived and survey for safety (yours and theirs). You might toss a pack of M&Ms or a protein bar at the nurses you either like or hope to bribe into being nice.

Sometimes you have time to take off your coat. Sometimes you enter running and do not stop until 12 ½ hours later when you sign out to go home. All the while, you are aware of the dangers, the position of the inmates in your building, and the string on your PPD.

The PPD is a personal protection device about the size of a garage door opener with a clip on one side to attach to your clothes, and a string hanging from the top. In an emergency, theory says that you will pull the string on the PPD, a light in the Control Center will indicate where you are, and several big strong folks with weapons will come to your aid. Fortunately, I never had to find out if it worked, but I knew as I walked the yard, especially alone at night, that little string was my lifeline.

There are tricks to staying safe. Never put an inmate between you and a door. Never allow an inmate to walk into the hall or an exam room until the CO has patted them down. Never examine an inmate in a closed room without someone else present, preferably someone bigger and stronger than you are.

Never leave an inmate alone in the exam room. If you step out of the exam room for a moment, he stands or sits in the hallway in view of the CO. Never share anything personal about yourself, like your full name, especially if you are as easy to find as I am. Information is currency, remember?

Maintaining the appropriate distance between you and inmates with one hand while practicing nursing with the other hand presents challenges. Always keeping one eye on the patient and the other visualizing an escape route, the life of a corrections nurse is complicated. Knowing which staff watches out for you, especially the COs, makes a world of difference. Those who like you have your back.

One CO, a sergeant who treated me like family, made a point to check in with me every day. He talked softly about family, and I think I reminded him of his mother or grandmother; both are good. The sergeant deployed somewhere out there with the military, and I hope someone has his six (is watching his back).

Another CO watched as I approached him, announcing over the radio that a nurse was on the walk. He gave me tips, like wearing something distinctive on my head in the winter because my navy blue scrubs and coat were hard to distinguish from the prisoners' dress blues. I knew those COs were watching over me, and the inmates were aware.

COs who are not fond of you will not perform their duties as expected, which could put you in danger. One CO failed to announce over the radio when I entered the yard. Telling the CO when you move between buildings means that he should inform the yard officers, via hand-held radio, to watch for you. That CO, who could not pull himself away from his computer and YouTube videos, left me unprotected until the COs on the walk, who kept a sharp eye at all times, saw me approach them. The yard COs are amazing.

The delinquent CO loved to use my full name with the inmates, though I requested that he used only *Nurse Jones*. Googling Sherry Jones Mayo, at that time, would lead you straight to my door, five miles from the prison. People are people, and some people are jerks. This same CO showed up in health care every day with a lunch box full of contraband that no one seemed ever to check.

Loophole?

~~~

Medical Clinic: What Happens in Prison Stays in Prison

Inmates receive appointments for various medical complaints. Rule of thumb says the prisoner has to see the nurse three times about the same complaint, unless it is emergent, before seeing the doctor. In some places, the docs avoid seeing patients, effectively turning care and responsibility back to the nurses. The ping-pong game between staff represents another power struggle and source of frustration for staff and inmates.

In addition to the daily appointments, divided among the nurses, are emergencies. A CO might call from a housing unit saying they were sending a patient with flu symptoms to us, which is usually not an emergency, and simply needs to run its course. On the other hand, a CO might call with a real emergency, which requires canceling standing appointments and rescheduling them. Inmates are never happy with those situations, although they feel differently when *they* are the emergency.

Inmates hurt each other and themselves. In those cases, the nurses drop everything and run with a jump kit and a wheelchair to the location of the sick or injured patient. Those situations have the potential to try the nurses' patience or tug on their heartstrings.

Rarely do we find humor in those circumstances. However, watching one of the nurses visibly stifling the urge to vomit, while pushing a puking patient through the yard, was funny. Sorry, Vetra* ... we all have our weaknesses.

The interactions between staff, and between inmates and staff, can provide immense entertainment. Like the nurse who wore her pants like hip-huggers, revealing butt cleavage. She loved to lean over the desk of the CO and giggle as they watched YouTube videos together. More SMH (shake my head) than entertaining, we rubbernecked her antics as one watches a car accident.

Another nurse was angry with everyone. In her eyes, everything was BS. Every complaint was unfounded, every phone call unnecessary. Her goal in life was to avoid work, and she spent much of each shift hiding, often napping, in unused rooms.

She constantly ate, though I never understood how she managed to smuggle in so much food. She also took 2-3 hour lunches, leaving her work for the other nurses. Rumor was that she had a friend in high places.

One fabulously entertaining nurse smuggled entire Chinese dinners. She shoved the polystyrene containers down the front and back of her scrubs and held her scrub jacket tightly around her belly with one hand. At the gate, she whispered to the officer, "Here is my coat but don't make me take off my smock." CO: "Food?" RN: "Yep." Most of us did not attempt anything of that magnitude, but the thought of that nurse, pulling container after container out of her britches, still makes me laugh.

Most of us stuck together, worked as a team, and enjoyed our jobs. Doing the impossible in corrections is like doing the impossible on the road as a medic or in the ER as a trauma nurse. You gain immense satisfaction and veer away from compassion fatigue when your work makes a difference. Nevertheless, the pendulum swung widely from one inmate to the next, one staff to the next, one day to the next.

When we had a moment, we kibitzed about some of our fonder or funnier clinic calls, marveling that people could do such things to each other or themselves. We wondered how men covered in tattoos balked at their annual tuberculin skin test (*very* small needle). To buoy one another and keep our sanity, we laughed and wished we could tell all. We cannot tell everything, but the following pages contain our thoughts and feelings about some things that happened working in the medical clinic.

~~~

Inmate: "I lost 8 pounds!"
RN: "Did you mean to?"
Inmate: "No, not really."
RN: "If you were a girl, you would be overjoyed!"
Inmate (Referring to other male prisoners): "We have enough of those in here already."

Of course, he was right. Tattooed eyebrows, ponytails in scrunchies, and insistence upon feminine identifiers of *miss* or *ma'am* surrounded us in a male-populated prison. Some assume a woman's persona after living for years as a straight man. Some become *gay for the stay*.

One lovely nurse, oozing with charm and speaking with a lilting southern accent, greeted these *ladies* with poise and style. She would say, "Miss Cannon* you are looking beautiful today," commenting on glowing skin or a new hairdo. The Southern nurse might slip some *ladies* a packet of triple antibiotic ointment, also known as liquid gold, during med lines. Was it a nursing treatment for chapped lips or a way for a girl to look her shiny-lipped best? You decide.

~~~

Radiology Tech: "Here are your callout's (patient's) films."
RN: "Seriously? Again? GAWD! How many things can you shove down your penis before you figure out that's not a good idea?"

For some inmates, setting aside the obvious mental health issues, shoving things where they do not belong often accomplishes the primary goal of every prisoner: Get out. Get off the grounds to an all-you-can-eat place with good drugs and pretty nurses. Become the center of attention as the diversion provides twisted entertainment.

Libby tells me about the joy of reviewing films with the radiology (x-ray) technician before seeing the patient. Not everyone with improperly placed objects, whether in the penis, rectum, or digestive tract, left the grounds for an ER visit. If the objects posed no immediate problem, many stayed where they were. Much to the inmates' dismay, ingested items only earned a small cup of Milk of Magnesia (MoM) to encourage passing the items out of the body the old-fashioned way.

Inmates love to swallow batteries. Usually, the batteries were small, new (no corrosion), and unless large enough in number to create a bowel obstruction, left to pass on their own with Magic MoM. Libby remembers one overachiever who swallowed 18 D-cell batteries, the kind used for large flashlights. I have to wonder how the inmate procured the fancy feast, and if those huge batteries were hard to wash down.

~~~

Inmate: "Nurse, I just want you to know I got your back. If anything goes down, they gonna think you one of us, cause nobody will hurt you."

Nurses in corrections often try to be Sweden, neutral, non-judgmental, giving medical and mental health care without adding insult to injury for an incarcerated patient. Like the COs, we try to do our jobs while remaining firm, fair, and consistent. *Freddy had prior run-ins with Nurse Smith when she was new, establishing that the nurse was a visitor in the inmates house, so this position of protection was a huge leap in expressing trust and respect. Here is the back-story.

Inmates receive medications up to three times a day. If the prisoner is in segregation (seg), the medication comes to his door. The prisoners in the general population (GP) line up at the med room window.

Those *med lines* sometimes suffer delays, cutting into the inmates' yard or personal time. The easiest person to blame for delays is the nurse, and inmates are wont to point fingers away from themselves, and focus on offenses against them. *Not my fault* represents a larger societal issue, but this is prison, not The World.

After one huge fit of anger during a delayed med line, Freddy stomped away, cursing, without his evening medications. Later, Freddy came back to the window as the nurse was cleaning up and asked to talk. Inmates give nurses kites (written requests to see the doctor, etc.) at those times, and often relay requests and concerns they cannot express in front of others. The nurse went to the window, the two hashed out their differences, came to an understanding, and Freddy went back to his cell.

The next day, in front of other inmates and the second nurse, Freddy apologized. He finally figured out Nurse Smith was one of the few people who had his back, medically, and he wanted to let her know he respected her. Apologies are huge, respect is everything, and although the danger is always present, staff rarely receives a public apology from an inmate. It was Nurse Smith's first inmate apology, and she admits it gave her goosebumps.

~~~

Staff: "I do not know if anybody is interested, but off the top of my head, I wrote down some of the things inmates either stuck somewhere or swallowed recently. Most of these guys went by car to the hospital. Our tax dollars at work."

Libby's list was impressive. "Things stuck into the urethra: toenail clippers, paperclips folded into a fishhook, copper wire from an outlet shaped (and sized) like a hot dog, pens. Things swallowed: fluorescent light bulbs, zippers, razors, socks, lag bolt, toothbrush, and a Spork."

Creativity blossomed as the list continued. "Wires and other sharp objects stuck into the abdomen. A Spork in the knee and through the jaw. A razor was hidden in the hem of an inmate's shorts."

I can identify with the list and have seen many of those abuses and injuries. The line blurs between trauma, corrections, and psychiatric nursing. Nursing and treating those injuries in corrections is distinctively different. The tools are primitive and always locked up, the staff shortages more intense, and the dangers to nursing staff far greater than at any inner city hospital.

Responding to an emergency with a wheelchair and jump bag, two nurses look almost comical as they run down the sidewalk. In the winter, they push through slush, ice, and snow. In summer, sweat pours down their faces as they travel to the farthest points of the grounds.

In all weather, they wonder what they will find. They wonder if the complaint is a set-up to divert attention away from two nurses with sharps and drugs, running through a walkway crowded with inmates who will not move. Any one or two of those inmates could take a nurse out in seconds in those close quarters. Serious injury or death is always possible for nurses responding to care for an injured prisoner.

~~~

RN: "The CO from 8 Block called. Mr. Green* is throwing up blood again. They said he was too weak to walk over here. I will get the chair if somebody comes with me."

The nurses moved the chair to 8 Block, one pushing and one pulling, uphill, through snow and patchy ice, to retrieve Mr. Green. They found him sitting halfway up a stairwell (at least he was not face down wedged between the toilet and a bunk). The CO pointed to a plastic bag near him where he was throwing up "blood," which looked like fecal matter (stool) to the nurses.

Pushing Mr. Green into the exam room, one of the nurses asked the doctor to see the patient. Mr. Green had a severely distended abdomen and complained of 12 / 10 pain (no one stops at 10 on a 1-10 scale). The doctor refused, said to give the inmate some Maalox and MoM, and send him back to the cellblock. Welcome to the sock hop; remove your shoes and prepare to boogie as responsibility lobs between staff members.

Management got involved, the dance changed partners a few times, and finally the primary nurse acquired a test strip designed to test fecal matter for blood. She obtained a positive reading, the doctor huffed, puffed, and blamed everyone for the price of tea in China, and the patient went to the ER. Unlike in The World, corrections doctors do not trust nursing judgment, especially if it means more paperwork. After the incident, the doctor wrote a formal complaint against the nurse for failing to use the words he would have chosen in the transfer paperwork. Welcome to Corrections, where folks do not get mad, they get even.

~~~

CO: "Ok, look at that. Is it blood, or Kool-Aid, or chocolate, or what?"

The two nurses stepped into the single segregation cell containing nothing except a plastic covered mattress and the normal hardware. Seasoned paramedics before becoming nurses, they surveyed the scene.

Manny began, "The middle of the puddle has partially digested food. Outside of that circle is a dark red liquid that splatters up onto the walls, which took some force. If the inmate just poured blood saved from another injury, or if it is not blood, he could not have reproduced that spatter pattern on the wall. And the color is perfect for blood."

The nurses looked at one another, nodded in agreement, and told the CO that without test strips, which they did not have; they could not state beyond any doubt that it was blood. However, from their professional perspectives and experience, the inmate, who claimed to have swallowed razor blades, did throw up blood. The officer should send the inmate to the health care nurses, who would likely ship him to the hospital.

The CO said, "Oh, crap" because he would need a sergeant from Control to move the patient from seg to health care. The nurses nodded and smiled. When they got far enough from the cells that no one could hear them, they giggled. "Sleuthing at its best; that was freaking fun."

~~~

CO: (On the phone) "I am bringing you a cutter. He sliced his arms up good this time. I will meet you in the ER."

Unless the bleeding is uncontrolled, doctors' stitch on site during the day, and at night, the inmate goes to an ER. Cutters often refuse sutures or an ER trip for minor injuries. If we can control their bleeding with Steri-strips (thin pieces of medical tape), we can usually talk the inmate into allowing us to tape up the wounds, even if the inmate removes the tape as soon as he returns to segregation.

One night, while the nurse was cleaning a cutter's wounds and preparing to close them, the CO made a comment about the stupidity of cutting. The nurse said that sometimes people cut because it provides a different kind of pain. Cutting takes people away from something in their minds or memories they cannot consciously escape. Uncharacteristically, the inmate spoke. He usually sat silently while people talked about him.

"She's right. When I was little, I was sexually abused. No matter what I do, I cannot forget it, and sometimes the memories are worse than being in this prison. If I cut, I can quiet the memories down for a while." Unlike most abused children, this inmate had not become an abuser but used and sold drugs in The World to deal with his past.

The CO let his guard down just long enough to look at my patient and see what I saw, a little boy hurt by adults. That little boy never grew up, never got over the abuses, and in later years, used drugs to try to escape the memories. The world failed to protect him as a boy and then made fun of his coping strategies as an adult. The CO would deny it, but I swear I saw his eyes well up with tears.

~~~

Radiology Tech: "Middle-aged inmate got his behind handed to him in the housing unit, so the doctor ordered some films to check for broken bones. The inmate's face and shirt were all bloody, and as I positioned him on the x-ray table, I noticed 'THUG LIFE' tattooed across the front of his neck. The inmate started whimpering like a hurt puppy and said how much it hurt. I turned my head toward him and asked, 'What hurts, the THUG LIFE?'"

~~~

RN: "Oh, God, that's all you got? Put that nasty thing away."

For some reason, the male's inclination to display what he was born with, and what he can do with it, intensifies when incarcerated. In the ER, we examined genitals to assess illness or injury or to place a Foley catheter to drain the bladder. In prison, some of the boys like to get naked, jump on a table, and show you their junk.

Inmates do not need a reason to *whip it out* randomly as you walk by their cells or go into their exam rooms. They watch you walk down the hall and stare as though immersed in a porn flick. Because the eyes follow us wherever we go, no matter how desperately uncomfortable we might become on hot days, we always wear a jacket to hide our behinds. Well, all of us except for the nurse who wore her scrubs around her hips. She never understood why she got so much negative attention.

~~~

Staff: "I do not know if inmates have the need to hurt themselves, or if they just want to do something to get out of jail for a while. Several with abdominal wounds will reopen the sutures to go back to the hospital, often smiling because they found a way to go back to a soft bed and waiters in scrubs (nurses). One guy went so far as to pull his intestines out, and another cut his intestines open so he could spray fecal matter at staff. I remember another inmate chewing the leather restraints off and then chewing his wrists. I just do not get it."

~~~

CO: (Over the radio) "Nurses respond to Housing Unit 12 NOW, we have an emergency."

Without any indication of the nature of the emergency, two nurses grabbed the large jump kit and ran to the housing unit. Upon arrival, they found an inmate on the floor with his head fairly well bashed in by his Bunkie (roommate). It seems the injured man talked too much.

The talker did not respect his Bunkie's pleas for silence. Feeling disrespected, the Bunkie stomped on the man's head until the talking stopped. The inmate with the flattened head left the prison by ambulance and later died from his injuries.

~~~

CO: "Can I bring *Luke up to the exam room? He would not let anyone look at his bandages all day, but he said he would let you. I guess he did not like the day shift nurse, though I cannot say as I blame him."

Luke went into segregation following his episode of self-mutilation and refused twice-daily wound checks from all but a few nurses. That night, the COs brought Luke in chains to the exam room, barefoot, and wearing only a Gumby suit. I took his vital signs.

One of the COs in the room told Luke he needed to "stop that cutting shit" and asked Luke to promise never to do it again. Luke said he could not make that promise, and to his credit, Luke always kept his word. After a few minutes of conversation, I asked Luke to promise *me* that for 24 hours he would not hurt himself. Just give me 24 hours.

Luke thought about it, looked away from me, and asked the officers, "If I give something up will you take it and not write me a ticket?" The COs laughed knowing Luke had nothing in the cell. He asked again, and they agreed. Luke turned to me, made the promise, and opened his mouth.

He had hidden several razor blades under his tongue. The CO removed the razor blades and kept his bargain. Luke did not cut again for several months.

~~~

RN: "Mama Jones, we are going to have a good day today. No matter what happens, we are going to have a good day. Ok?"

I loved working with Vetra. She was hilariously funny (coined *Mangina*), and a good nurse who worked in jails before state prisons. She was a patient teacher, and always jumped in to help. She ran herself ragged, so I would sometimes slip a pop or candy bar into her pocket. My only regret is not taking notes as I heard her talking to prisoners, defusing tense situations with humor and empathy.

~~~

CO: (On the phone) "We got one over here that got cut pretty bad, can you bring a wheelchair and come and get him?"

Nurses arrived to find a CO holding pressure on an inmate's face, and a fair amount of blood on the floor around him. The man stared straight ahead. After the initial assessment of the wound, the nurses determined he could transport by wheelchair to the clinic for exam and orders. When the RN removed the paper toweling provided by the CO to examine the wound, it spurted blood, so the inmate held pressure while one nurse pushed his chair and another lugged the big jump kit.

The inmate said he did not know what happened or who did it. High-security inmates usually have an in-house justice system, and as this wound was across the face, it may have been a Do Not Snitch message. Whoever sliced did a good job, nicking an artery, and buying the inmate an ambulance trip off grounds for a few hours.

It could have been worse. After the inmate was packaged and shipped to the hospital, the COs called the clinic to report they found the weapon. The lid from a #10 can still held the chunk of flesh the assailant dug out of the inmate's cheek.

~~~

CO: (On the radio) "Need a nurse to cellblock 4, please; right away." (Phone call) "We got a prisoner stabbed in the neck in building four, and the CO is holding pressure. It was spurting, and he lost a lot of blood."

Lugging the large jump kit, three nurses responded. Spurting means artery, neck artery means possible fatality if not controlled. Of the three nurses responding, one had no prior nursing experience before prison, one had some hospital experience, and one was a trauma nurse. They arrived to find the inmate flat on the floor, laying in a large pool of blood, with a CO holding pressure to his neck.

The two less experienced nurses, Lucy and Ethel started going through the jump kit, looking for and pulling out supplies. The trauma nurse, Mary, dove into the blood and assessed the inmate. He was lucid and responded appropriately, so Mary asked somebody to spike a line and give her the IV start kit while she looked for a vein. Lucy spiked a small bag (should have been large), unnecessarily pouring saline on the floor as she bled the line (got rid of air bubbles) while Ethel tried to shove an oxygen tank between Mary and the patient.

Mary directed Ethel to the other side of the patient and asked her to apply a non-rebreather mask, turning the oxygen all the way up. Lucy handed Mary the spiked tube, and Mary inserted the IV catheter, first try, no tourniquet. As she taped it down, Mary thought, "Cool … I haven't lost my touch, and I still rock."

A CO appeared over Mary's shoulder and took pictures. The inmate smiled broadly for the camera. They all laughed. In a difficult situation, the nurses had a save.

Lucy wrote up the report as though she were the primary nurse, assisted by Ethel and Mary. They finished the shift, stopping at Control with the signed reports. Another day's pay earned, they punched the time clock and went home.

Mary felt a sense of accomplishment, just like the old trauma days. The icing on the cake came later in the clinic. In a waiting room full of inmates lining up for medications, one yelled out for Mary.

"Hey. I remember you. I saw you on the floor with that guy. You got down in that blood, and you took care of business. That's why they hired you, cuz you good with that stuff."

Mary yelled back, "Yep. That's why they hired me. I am good at that stuff. " Validation, appreciation, respect.

~~~

What is on Your "Top 10" List?

The last time I connected socially with my corrections peeps, we talked about some of our prison memories. There are things we will never forget. Whether the answer to *what is on your top 10 list* represented their most or least liked items, here they are. You can decide whether they are love or loathe entries.

- Seeing your favorite coworkers sitting at the desk laughing (instead of frantically running around)

- Attention seeking behaviors, which are 99% BS manipulations

- COs rewarding porters with real coffee at the end of shift

- COs who think other staff wants to sleep with them

- Coworkers pulling together in emergencies

- Cussing inmates out (in a good way) when they do stupid things
- Dressing changes, especially twice daily
- Every door (including the bathroom) and all supplies locked up
- Everyone has a nickname (like the RN, "Evilene")
- Exposure to infectious diseases and blood borne pathogens
- Fake bleeding, fake complaints, drama
- Finding a candy bar you forgot was in your stash
- Getting in the car wearing scrubs and shoes from work: *ick* factor
- Giving inmates tips for getting back out in into The World
- Graduating from the Academy and getting hired
- Hearing, "You care about us, don't you?"
- Ice cold Diet Coke/Mountain Dew from the pop machine
- Inmates believing there are no restrictions on how they talk to you
- Inmates diverting wound care medical tape to make shanks
- Inmates injuring themselves, then demanding wound care
- Inmates selling food for hits of coffee
- Inmates telling each other to stop harassing a nurse because she might "Go all Detroit on your ass; she's from the East Side."
- Inmates who play Burger King with their medications ("I want this one, I don't want that one …")
- Inmates: "I can't pee, will you Cath me?" (Tube to empty bladder)
- Knowing the CO has my back
- Lack of, or outdated supplies and equipment
- Laughing at the most insane stuff without worrying about PC
- Making a difference in people's lives; ALL people
- Manipulative behavior like hunger strikes

- Masturbation, masturbation, masturbation
- Muzzleloading pens, staples, and paper clips (shaping them like a fish hook so they will not come out)
- No cell phone for 12 hours unless you run out to your car
- Nurses moving *their* inmates with complicated treatments, smelly bandage changes, or bad attitudes over to *your* callout list
- Outdated technology, not enough working computers
- Penises *everywhere;* "I have seen too many penises."
- Prisoners cheeking their medications (hiding pills in the mouth between cheek and gums to sell, snort, or save for later)
- Prisoners dropping their eyes and, preparing to confess something, saying, "Nurse, you're gonna be mad."
- Prisoners flinging urine, feces, and semen at you
- Realizing some prisoners are just bad, and you cannot save them
- Receiving respectful treatment from co-workers and inmates
- Recognition as finalist for Employee of the Year
- Remembering that some inmates were abused or neglected, mothers left them, no strong figures to teach and lead them; not to excuse them, but knowing the back story helps with communication
- Responding to an unknown medical to find someone with whom you established professional rapport has completed suicide
- Reviewing amusing stories that you cannot repeat to outsiders
- Rumors, rumors, rumors
- Satisfaction of doing the impossible
- Seg inmates putting their face close to the chuck hole to get staff to lean in, then flinging bodily fluids through the opening
- Staff ransacking your stuff and stealing your food and pens

- Staff slapping the backs of inmates heads (or the backs of their hands) like their Mamas *should* have done

- Staff who rile up the inmates

- Unknown medical: Finding an inmate brutally beaten or murdered

- Using prison language back at inmates: no PC

- Watching a prisoner die for the first time; staff couldn't save him

- Watching officers getting Taser qualified

- When an inmate delivers a heartfelt apology

~~~

Active Shooter; Active Shooter; Active Shooter

Beautiful sunny day, working the 1100 - 2330 shift, brought coffee to my favorite front desk CO, cleared the gate, and stood in front of my friends, the pop and junk food machines. With a coat pocket full of singles and change, I loaded up with Mountain Dew for Vetra, Diet Coke for me, and bribery treats for Nurse Cranky Pants. With my coat over my arm, I was about to turn and head for the door to the yard when I heard the overhead announcement: "Active shooter, active shooter, active shooter."

Before I could cognitively register the words, I found my body had dropped to the floor, and plastered against a concrete-block pony wall next to the junk machines. I peeked through windows above the wall into the gate. Walking from Control into the secure gate area was an African American male, about 6' 7" tall, dressed in black that covered all but his eyes, and carrying a rifle as tall as me.

Grateful for training and road smarts that kicked in before I had a chance to think, I looked around. The adrenaline rush from this completely new situation prevented breaking any body parts when I hit the floor, so I thought about an escape route or hiding place. There was an office tucked away next to the machines.

The open door was large, metal, and contained a lock. The woman inside the office, a supervisor, sat nonchalantly at her desk. She looked at me, and I asked, "What do we do now" hoping that she would invite me to her safe place and lock the door. She shrugged, said, "I have no idea; it would have been nice to be trained for this."

I peeked back over the pony wall and saw that the shooter was gone. The only places he could go were the visitors and training areas, over to another yard separate from mine, or outside to leave the compound. Seeing an opportunity to speak with Control, 20 feet away, I asked what I should do. They told me to go on to my work area, buzzing open the next Sally Port to get into the yard.

Because the Control Center officer told me to walk in an open area, I hoped this was a drill. Scanning the grounds, I saw that no one was on the walkway except me, so apparently everyone had already taken cover. If this were an actual, Control could have sent me to medical knowing every nurse would deploy from there, so I walked very quickly to the medical building. I do not think I have ever felt more vulnerable.

I went into medical and saw the entire staff in the waiting room, chairs in a circle, chatting. They were in front of an open window, laughing, eating snacks, with their radios in pockets or next to them on the floor. I said, "Drill, right?" They were not sure but suspected as much.

Anxious to learn how to handle things in the event of an actual event, I asked questions of the person in charge (the doctor). He had no idea. I asked the charge nurse about how we should respond. She said I was in Group A with Jan, Joe, Sally, Mark, and Tom, the doctor. We would deploy first in case anything happened, but there was no plan.

I went to the back for a moment to stuff my pockets with gloves, and a few emergency tools from my personal stash. There was still no formal notification that this was a drill. Too many years with military, paramilitary, law enforcement, and emergency management, perhaps, but I wanted to be prepared, and was happy to play.

Time went on, people continued to chat, snack, and laugh, and after the exercise had ended, folks returned to duty. We rescheduled clinic appointments and dealt with rowdy, upset inmates. We ran around trying to make up time distributing medications and treatments.

I have two takeaways from that experience. First, never miss an opportunity to practice procedures and skills that might save lives, especially your own. Second, what my old EMT instructor Jon Beem pounded into my head was true. Some things become part of your autopilot, and you will switch to that mode when you need it. Like when someone announces, "Active shooter, active shooter, active shooter."

Pre-Prisoner Health Care: Not Your Average Patient

Working with those who find themselves on the wrong side of the cuffs began long before I worked in a state prison. As a road paramedic, I transported many pseudo-seizures, also known as get-out-of-jail-free incidents, to the local ERs. Then as a trauma nurse, I received many of those patients. We have several tests for determining if someone is faking a seizure. Those who can bear a vigorous sternal rub, penlight to the base of the thumbnail, or orbital notch pressure without flinching often fail the final determination between real and faked seizures.

Some folks use a standard test that has survived generations of EMTs transporting incarcerated patients from jails to ERs. Elevate the patient's arm over the head as they are laying on the cot and drop it over the face. The hand and arm will miraculously move to the side, avoiding causing injury, if the person is conscious and faking seizure. If the patient is not faking, you may deliver to the local ER a seizure patient with a nosebleed. Oops, good thing PD takes pictures before transport.

~~~

As staff members within the hospital emergency departments, especially in the larger cities, we welcomed many patients in handcuffs escorted by uniformed officers. Those officers witnessed our blood draws as a course of legal procedure. Contrary to Internet claims, we did not use the largest bore needle possible, or purposely miss several times before hitting a vein. No one has time for that.

A handcuffed patient with an armed officer escort in the hospital can be disconcerting for some nurses. The inconveniences of starting an IV on a cuffed arm, or assisting with toileting, as we do not want to touch *that* to put *it* into a urinal, are obvious. We get through it.

Nonetheless, I never understood why nurses feared working with prisoners. You should worry about the *other* patients who can become violent and wail on you with four free limbs, not the person tethered to the bed with an armed officer sitting beside him. On a short-stay unit, every prisoner admitted became my patient, much to the relief of my coworkers.

Cuffed patients admitted to the hospital were often calm, respectful, and appreciated any kindness shown to them. Remember the uniformed officer with a sidearm, pepper spray, or Taser sitting next to the bed? He totally has this. Though he asks nothing of you, giving a cop an occasional cup of coffee makes his stay easier, too.

~~~

Detained patients in the ER are a different story. Often the officer escorts the EMS transport with the patient cuffed to a gurney. Prime time for these folks is weekends, during a full moon, following a sports competition, or after the bars close. Loud, aggressive patients, not always male, come in ready to challenge everyone within earshot. Transferring those patients to an ER stretcher often takes several strong warm bodies.

If the patient is under arrest, the officer stays. If the officer needs only to witness the blood draw, he does not have to stay and watch (or smell) the offender. If LEOs (law enforcement officers) leave and take their cuffs, we can replace those cuffs with restraints. The paperwork sucks, but patient safety is a priority.

Wrestling with an intoxicated patient spouting verbal threats and attempting intimidation can be entertaining to watch. If only video-taping new nurses attempting to *reason* with those folks, and gently asking for their cooperation, were legal. The play by play would be priceless as the intoxicated persons' limbs move independently of one another, each with different intent. LEOs and experienced RNs exchange knowing looks and turn their heads away momentarily to break character and laugh.

Some of the things people say and do when intoxicated are funny. Alcohol is a social lubricant that bypasses the sober person's cognitive filters and controls. One intervention we administer is moving cell phones out of reach to prevent drunk dialing/drunk texting. Unfortunately, unless folks are restrained, we cannot prevent them from removing their clothes. Being drunk and naked go together like peanut butter and jelly.

Moreover, they pee on themselves. Those who are barely conscious require precautions like the insertion of a Foley catheter (tube into the bladder), and sometimes a nasal trumpet (tube into their nose to guarantee their airway and breathing). We monitor them, keep them alive, and hope they will sleep off the intoxication. Dim the lights, tuck them in, say nighty-night, and bring the officer a cup of coffee.

Sometimes folks revert to a more sensitive nature or time in their lives (acting like five years old), and openly weep to the officer or nurse at the bedside. Drunk crying is sloppy and self-pitying, which does not encourage the engagement of our empathetic genes. Serious situations, like when the drunk driver causes a fatality and expresses concern about possible incarceration, brings out the tough-love gene, and our therapeutic conversation can be sobering. Wrong audience for a pity party, dude.

~~~

RN: Lou is an ICU nurse baffled by cuffed patients.

"There's nothing like coming into the room first thing in the morning, and finding your unconscious, intubated patient cuffed to the bed. Even though I understand the precautions, it just always seemed unnecessary to have them chemically *and* physically restrained."

~~~

Medic: Andy tells me about the old days when pepper spray was new.

"A police officer used his pepper spray generously on a couple of young males involved in a fight. Not a big deal. We transported them to the local hospital for treatment.

"We were still there doing reports when we heard them both start screaming. Come to find out they were at the sink washing off the pepper spray. It ran down their chests and made its way to their, um, 'sensitive parts.' I'm sure it didn't feel good. That one still makes me laugh."

Andy shares another law enforcement encounter that makes him giggle. I guess if you are a male, anywhere is a potential bathroom. When you gotta go, you gotta go.

"We were working in the South End of the city. The officer was trying to get a drunk to cooperate. As we were walking the drunk to our ambulance, he whipped it out and started urinating in the middle of the street in broad daylight. The surprised officer yelled, calling attention to the drunk in case anyone did not see him, 'Put that thing away!'"

~~~

RN: Cheryl works in the ER and loves dealing with LEOs.

"Cops and ER nurses have an affinity for one another and shared language. They become friends partly because they understand some of each other's worlds and challenges. I love to see officers in the ER when they bring patients into my section. For that period, even though I have to deal with someone who may be less than desirable as a patient, I feel safe.

"I love watching the officers watch me handle the situations that invariably arise when you deal with someone who is insanely drunk. The officer will stand back, fold his arms, and smile because he knows he is going to be entertained for a little while. Unlike the impatience officers may have with inexperienced nurses, they know seasoned old women like me can handle anything, and will not take crap from the disrespectful out-of-control drunks. We do not abuse them, but we do not let them run us either. Cops love that."

~~~

Medic: Rhys recalls accepting custody of a patient after police Tasing.

"My partner Chris and I transported a patient the cops Tased. He had two embedded Taser prongs that we couldn't remove. The first was at the top of the head, and the other in his butt cheek.

"On the way to the ER, the patient starts flicking the prong stuck in his head. Overheard in a taped radio line is my voice describing my transport of a suspect who had been 'unicorned,' and me telling him to 'quit flicking that thing. It's in your brain. You'll forget math or something.'"

~~~

RN/Medic: Nurse Coop tells of one officer busting a patient *in* the ER.

"Dude was rolled into trauma after being hit by a car. He was not hurt badly, but as medics brought him in, he was threatening to sue the driver, the paramedics, and the ER staff before he was off the ambulance gurney. As we are wheeling him to CT scan, a bike cop walks up to the stretcher.

"Right about the time the patient is threatening to sue the cop, too, the cop drops a jaywalking ticket right on the guy's chest. The look on the patient's face as his lawsuit threat got shot down was priceless. It was a scream.

"We would have loved to share high-fives all around, but the trauma surgeon, Dr. Darth Vader, was working that day. He was old school, large ego, and no sense of humor. We got a lot of mileage out of the story in the breakroom, though. We do not always get to witness real-time Karma, but we did that night."

~~~

RN: Bunny tells us about a *Get out of Jail Free* card.

"A couple of months ago, we got a patient from a nearby city's police department with the diagnosis of incarceritis. When the other inmates saw him leave, they all magically got incarceritis, too. The funniest part was watching the cops try to watch all the prisoners that came to the ER. They had to run from one to the next to keep an eye on them all."

~~~

We agree that whether our history is on the streets, in the ER, or in corrections, the experiences change our worldview. We become more like helicopter parents, hovering over our children, watching more closely over their television and Internet choices. We are stricter, do not threaten, and follow through consistently with punishments and rewards as fairly as we are able. We worry more, show it less, love without embarrassment, and know that the last time we see someone may be the last time we see them. We say I love you a lot.

We worry about who we friend on social media, who tags us in their pictures, who posts to our timeline, who knows our real names, who sees our family pictures, and who knows our personal information. We *pat down* constantly for our keys, thinking every door we pass through, including the bathroom, requires unlocking for entry. We listen to the noises outside our homes at night, wondering if someone is looking in, fleetingly entertaining thoughts about those inmates who promised to 'look us up' when released.

Some of us are vague about where we work. Libby decided to "put it out there right away" and deal with the fallout. She says, "It takes a special person to make it in corrections. Between the inmates and the environment, you need to be able to adapt." Now I understand why so many people, inmates, COs and medical staff, used to smile and say, "Oh, Nurse Jones, you fit right in here." It was a compliment.

I do not think I have ever been more comfortable in a job. The years on the road as a medic, in the ER as a trauma nurse, and in a closed psychiatric unit, all worked together to give me the skills for corrections. I miss it. I wonder if *the boys* are making progress, learning what they need to know to survive in The World when they parole or complete their sentences. I wonder if anyone is bringing the porters post-shift coffee.

When you are born in Detroit, you sometimes keep some of the rough edges and wear them as a badge of honor. I appreciate my formal education, yet realize life holds lessons you cannot find in books. The product of a hard-working, blue-collar, immigrant family, I can sit with princesses, ponder life with academics, and still roll with my ER and corrections homies. Wisdom and engaging with certain folks involves empathy, a servant heart, and living a transparent and authentic life. I try.

Prison taught me things about life, about other people, about myself. Putting judgment away and practicing nursing without bias took effort. Having a positive effect on people who did things that were too horrible to think about happened with intention.

When I stepped into the yard to begin my workday, I had to put all of the judgment, rationalization, and inner moral compass that threatened to condemn others away. If I did not, I would have taken it back home with me at the end of my shift. Therefore, when I turned in my PPD at the end of the day, the prison nurse persona went with it. Nurse Jones punched out and turned in her keys, and Sherry Jones Mayo got in the car to go home to her husband and cats.

<table>
<tr>
<td>

5

</td>
<td>

After the Call
When it Isn't Really *Over*

</td>
</tr>
</table>

There is an inviolability in a Critical Incident Stress Debriefing. What you say in the room stays in the room. However, we tell folks before the debriefing begins that they are welcome to share their words and experiences with those close to them after the meeting.

Julia, a woman in her forties, wanted her experience with loss and the crisis interventions that followed shared with others. She has asked me to tell her story so that others might know not only of the value of peer crisis intervention but also of the closeness with her best friend, Marie. The circumstances that led up to the debriefing and a small peek into the debriefing room, follow.

Julia's Story

Julia* was abused as a child. She never really talked about it much (or in detail) because she did not have many people close to her. Those to whom she confided heard stories that had the potential to make them a little uncomfortable.

Folks heard first-hand the kind of information we read about or see on TV or in movies. We do not want to be face-to-face with the pain of the person who suffered such unspeakable things. The violated person's agony is palpable, and it usually causes others to find someone a little more upbeat with whom to hang around. Someone with less drama.

Because of that, Julia did not have many close friends. In her adulthood, she found Marie,* a woman who had borne her share of pain and indignity. Marie could see through Julia's hurting to the true spirit beneath, the wounded child in an adult form who was still able to give and receive love.

Julia and Marie met through a volunteer organization that performs search and rescue operations and deploys through the United States Air Force. The friends spent time together preparing and training for ES

(Emergency Services) support positions. Marie was an accomplished scanner/observer who never quite convinced Julia to take aircrew training.

Julia was a *ground pounder* (ES worker who performs duties on the ground instead of in the air), although she greatly admired Marie's ability to serve from above. They shared a love of flying from different perspectives, with Marie looking down and Julia looking up. They both took great pride in their jobs and did them well. In addition to being her best friend, Marie was Julia's hero.

It was August. An aircrew from Julia's squadron participated in an Air Force assigned mission, searching for a teenaged boy who had been on a fishing trip in the mountains, and was reported overdue by his family. The pilot in command was instrument-rated commercial (single and multi-engine land and sea airplane), with more than 1,800 hours of flight time logged, and qualified for specialized mountain flying.

Sitting second seat was Marie, an accomplished observer, who also held ratings as scanner and skills evaluator. In the back seat of the Cessna 182 were a scanner trainee and expert military pilot. Their aircraft crashed into a mountain while performing their assigned mission, killing all three people aboard. The teenaged boy overdue from the fishing expedition was later found alive and well by other rescuers.

The organization to which Julia and Marie belonged had a CISM (Critical Incident Stress Management) plan in place to handle the emotional aftermath of trauma. A line of duty death (times three) would prove to be emotionally traumatizing for the remaining members, especially so for the families and close friends of those who died. While the strategic planning was set to facilitate the appropriate interventions, the hierarchy of the organization decided that their people did not need help. The CISM teams could not deploy.

Instead, phone calls to some of the members made by the CISM team offered support and education. The organization's command staff continued to maintain that the affected members did not need peer interventions. While the CISM team stood down, unable to make face-to-face contact, they continued the phone calls and redesigned strategies to accommodate the new plan of action. Local mental health folks became available to those emotionally wounded who would accept help. As expected, phone calls to those hurting from the aftermath of this trauma were a Band-Aid that would eventually tear open and reveal all the infection brewing beneath.

Three months later, a squadron commander, who was greatly concerned about the well-being of his members, again went through the chain of command requesting CISM interventions. The commander reported that his people were still hurting from the plane crash and line of duty deaths. He boldly rejected the earlier decision against deploying CISM, and once again requested the National Crisis Response Team. The squadron commander (Julia's friend DJ*) finally received approval for crisis intervention, and the plan abandoned three months before was set into place.

Holding a line of duty death intervention three months after a plane crash can be problematic. In addition to a delayed intervention, the team must also deal with the anniversary of the crash. The complexity of that situation requires deploying the most experienced and sensitive team members.

The well-meaning squadron commander, wanting to be thorough, invited to the debriefing the families of the deceased. He also invited the families of squadron members, muddying the purity and ease of a homogenous group. While that decision presented a challenge for the CISM team, it later turned out to be ideal. As the major issues were grief and loss, coming together helped to ease pain and increase cohesiveness.

Those who would come to the debriefing, expecting nothing, could leave with hope, some answers to their emotional dilemmas, and a personal plan of action aimed toward healing. Critical Incident Stress Debriefing (CISD) is a ritual of closure. These folks needed help getting to that point.

The supportive phone calls to Julia continued. Meanwhile, a complex strategic plan of action went into place to sustain the rest of the members, friends, and families of the members and victims. Julia's squadron commander, Dave Jones* (DJ) kept in touch with us by phone and email to let us know of his concern about Julia. He provided details about Julia's increasing grief and pain, and her disgust with her father's continued emotional abuse. DJ offered insights and observations regarding the folks around him.

DJ told us that he was with Julia when she found out she had lost her best friend. Julia had tearfully phoned her father, who told her to, "Get over it." Failing to gain comfort from her father, Julia walked toward DJ, who was waiting with open arms. A good friend, DJ, offered a comfort that Julia rarely allowed, as physical contact with other human beings was tentative and limited.

Julia sobbed uncontrollably for several minutes. When she finally spoke, she said something about really hating "that a—hole." DJ wondered what to do for Julia, who seemed trapped between those "Who are trying to make things better and one (her father) who enjoys making them worse. Where's the win?" Julia was, in DJ's eyes, a "very lost soul."

Three CISM peers had made calls to the members closest to those who died in the airplane crash. Those peers deployed to the mountainous region to offer some guidance and support for those still grieving. The CISM team included Chaplain Don, an ordained minister and paramedic from Texas, Dr. Mike, a hospice chaplain, psychologist, and ex-cop from California, and me, an ER trauma nurse/paramedic who recently moved from Detroit to Las Vegas.

We arranged for two local mental health professionals, Patty* and Joyce*, to join us at the site. Patty had been a part of the original CISM debriefing team for the local ES folks who responded to the airplane crash, and Joyce specialized in complicated PTSD (Post Traumatic Stress Disorder). We knew we were expecting a large group and wanted to balance the team as much as possible with not only male/female and Mental Health/Chaplain/ Peer, but also with those who held a variety of ES specialties.

The three peers wore enough hats to fill many of the requirements of the group. My husband kissed me goodbye at McCarron International with words of encouragement, knowing this would be an emotionally difficult intervention for everyone. While all five CISM team members were mobilizing to converge, I spent time on my long flight thinking about the phone calls with Julia and the emails we shared.

A few months before, when I first called Julia, I was unprepared for the conversation that transpired. I sat on my bedroom floor and only half-listened to her words while the other half of my brain prayed diligently for wisdom and guidance. I was not a mental health professional, not trained in counseling, but had dealt with people in crisis for many years from a nursing and peer perspective.

I could hear the anxiety in Julia's voice as she poured her heart out to a stranger. Julia had completed nursing school, though she did not spend much time in that profession. My being a nurse gave us a common bond that offered her comfort. I had not wanted to make that call, hoping one of the mental health folks, far more experienced than me in crisis intervention, would take on the assignment. All refused, stating that they were too far away "in case in turns out to be a critical situation."

So is it better to do nothing and leave this poor woman to her pain and solitude? The fact that the professionals with whom I was associated disowned this woman gave me the courage to step into a place possibly too deep for my level of training and experience. I figured that I could at least assess the situation and get the professionals moving as needed. Doing *nothing* was not an option.

While I listened and prayed, offering input that came more from my spirit than my brain, Julia and I spoke. The sun slowly set, the room grew dark, but I did not notice any of that until the call ended. My heart and soul were deeply engaged in the conversation with this woman who seemed to have lost everything and was without direction.

Her voice echoed in my head well into the night as I mentally reviewed the conversation, wondering what else I should have said. This was not a practice scenario where one may make mistakes. This was someone's life, and I took it and the relationship we had established very seriously.

I felt satisfied that we had done well with this first call, knowing that another call, or two, would follow. Then I would either refer Julia to mental health or send her on her way with another follow-up call later. As always, I reviewed the important parts of the conversation with Dr. Mike, who offered professional guidance and reassurance. What I lacked in education I made up for with instinct, and it usually served me well. Instincts are gifts, nothing about which I can take credit, but something for which I am deeply grateful.

A while later, Julia wrote to me, "I thought that I was doing really well with Marie's death, but today I realized that I was dying of a broken heart. She was all that I had, and I am having trouble living without her. I am not feeling suicidal, but I don't want to live either. I spoke to (the local mental health social worker) yesterday, and I don't believe that there is anything that she can do for me. I have nothing left to live for. (Marie) made my life worth living every day and now she is gone.

"Let me remind you again that I am not feeling suicidal. I just want to quit living. Please don't get anyone else involved in this matter. I will continue on the best that I can until Jesus calls me home."

I called Julia immediately after calling the suicide hotline local to her, ready with a name and number, and having forewarned their staff of the situation. Julia denied that she was suicidal, laughed at the thought, said she was saddened, but surely would not harm herself as her religion strictly prohibited such actions. She agreed to talk to the local mental health folks again.

We contracted during that phone call that Julia would not harm herself, that if she had any thoughts of harming herself, she would immediately call 911, the local mental health folks, or me. Julia said she was just not sleeping well, thought of Marie all the time, and was "just tired." She told me that her email reflected the desire to be in a place of no more pain, to sleep, and have some time of peace before facing yet another day without her best friend. Julia got through the night and the days that followed, but we kept in close contact.

I reminded Julia that she was on a roller coaster, and things would alternately get better and worse as she worked through her pain. I pleaded with her to maintain contact with the local mental health folks. Julia needed to know that I was not abandoning her, but her situation required a lot more than I could give. I was not local to her and wanted assurance that she was safe.

We talked about her value in this world, her lessons in this life, her goals for the future, and her plans to honor her best friend, Marie. Acknowledging that she was dealing with a broken heart, I shared some of my pain in life, assuring her that while I did not understand her specific grief and loss, I did know what it was like to feel pain, that it was indeed survivable. I called two more of my friends with the letters PsyD or PhD after their names for additional advice.

One of those friends, Dr. Joan, a certified thanatologist (grief specialist), told me that it was normal to want to "not live." "Since her grief is so intense right now, I think she should spend as much time as she can actively grieving." Joan did not advise to wallow in grief, as eventually we all tire of wallowing, but for Julia to go ahead and spend her time thinking about Marie. "Build a shrine. Assemble a scrapbook."

Joan told me to help Julia start looking for one tiny thing that might make her smile, like a chocolate ice cream cone. Eventually, the distractions, like talking about things that make her smile, would take more time than the wallowing, and things would start to look like they did before the loss. We tried it, Julia did tell me some positive things, and the conversations moved forward to a more healing type of exchange.

Phone conversations are not ideal for crisis intervention because you cannot read body language and facial expressions. If it is all that you have, it is better than walking away and saying you cannot do anything. I believe there is always a way. We can always do *something,* and we may have to be incredibly inventive.

Julia began to smile and laugh in those conversations. I saw the person that Marie saw and befriended. I felt hopeful that Julia would make it through her long, dark nights.

Snapping back to the moment, I realized I was through the first leg of my journey to the mountains, and soon arrived at the next airport. The second flight was on a puddle jumper from the international airport to a very small airport. After a loud and bumpy ride, I landed in a place I never heard of before and caught a shuttle to the hotel, arriving tired and hungry. Unfortunately, the hotel only had junk food machines, a great disappointment for weary travelers, so I grabbed a bag of peanut M&Ms and dropped my bags off in the room.

Don, Mike, and I had a brief conversation, mostly about our long trips from home and our empty stomachs. We agreed to meet the next morning over breakfast to strategize and review our materials. To be somewhat prepared for what may surface in a debriefing, it is best to have data about the folks who will be attending, the crash, those who died, what positions they held in the organization and so on.

To walk in unprepared is foolish, as there are always surprises in a debriefing. We just never know where or when they will arise. There is some level of comfort and direction for the CISM team in being as prepared as possible, so we did our homework.

Late that next afternoon DJ picked us up at the hotel, and we headed out to the debriefing location, which was also the squadron headquarters. We planned the Critical Incident Stress Debriefing (CISD) at the squadron on a regular meeting night, which assured maximum attendance. DJ also called folks personally to ensure their presence and expected upwards of 30 people: members of the rescue organization, their families, and the family members of the aircrew that perished in the crash.

The MHPs (Mental Health Professionals) arrived at the site shortly after Don, Mike and I. We met in a small room off to the side of the main meeting room to refine our strategy. There were many options available regarding how we would split the groups, so we discussed three separate plans. We determined that we would make a final decision of where to put whom as soon as the folks were on-site. We could ascertain what type of a group we had, how they interacted, and what debriefing strategy we would employ.

When the folks arrived, it became clear through conversations that this was a grief and loss situation. To split the attendees would be damaging to the continuity of the group, depriving them of the help they could offer one another in the grieving process. Since the group was so diverse, each team member was prepared to step in and redirect the conversation to a more productive dialogue in keeping with established goals.

After a short meeting to define the roles of each CISM team member, and specific signals we would use to communicate discretely with one another during the group meeting, we set the room up with the chairs in a large circle. We positioned our team members strategically around the room. As we spaced ourselves evenly within the circle, we each picked someone who might need our particular skills in communication. I sat next to Julia.

Patty was the team leader. She opened the group meeting, setting expectations. Patty reviewed the ground rules:

- This is not an operational critique

- It is not counseling but a structured discussion

- What we say in the room stays in the room

- No cell phones

- Once we begin, please stay for the whole meeting

- We are not going to take any breaks, but if you need to leave, go ahead, and know that a CISM team member will follow you to make sure you are ok, and then come back in the room with you

- If there is anyone who should not be in this room, please let us know

- We are only going to talk about "X" event

- Everyone should speak only for themselves, and from their perspectives

- No one has to talk if he or she does not want to

- The discussion format will go through seven phases, and so on

We went around the room introducing the team members. Acknowledgment came from some of the attendees as they recognized our names either from the conversations we had over the phone or from our positions within the organization. Some knew us, as soon as we began speaking, remembering the voices that reached out to them when they were hurting.

Patty and Joyce were the only outsiders to the organization, but they quickly gained acceptance and credibility because they were locals. It became clear to us almost immediately that the choices for the team members were right on target. Beginning the formal debriefing by going around the circle, Patty acknowledged the members and asked them to introduce themselves.

Because I can only share Julia's perspective, I will tell you that all who attended comforted her. The experiences of the other folks during the debriefing, what they felt and shared during our time together, were deeply personal. We honor their privacy.

Most debriefings begin with folks a little tentative about talking, which lessens as each begins to speak. The sharing increases as each member of the group gives a perspective that others find they have in common, putting aside that fallacy of uniqueness each may have originally conceived. They stop thinking, "I'm the only one who feels this way."

Some debriefings get a little deep in the feelings expression phase, especially in line of duty deaths, where emotions remain heightened, and the member's raw feelings about the situation persist. These open emotional wounds may continue to bleed profusely. The folks in these circumstances have had a limited time to heal, and they may still be trying to find a way to survive the all-consuming depth of their grief and sorrow.

There are moments when the emotion is not so heavy, and laughter erupts as folks recall and share memories of those who passed. Often it is a combination of both laughter and sorrow. A skilled leader addresses each person's perspective and concerns, and normalizes those reactions, helping each to see a path to healing.

In this particular debriefing, all was proceeding well and somewhat as predicted with only minor redirection until Julia spoke up. She provided that expected unexpected moment. The zinger from left field we anticipated, but had no idea about what it might contain, or who might fling it into the middle of the room.

We had pondered situations based upon who was in attendance and the conversations we had with folks before the debriefing started, but this confession caught us off guard. We anticipated something coming from other members, such as the family of the deceased pilot, those with whom there may have been conflict within the organization, or possibly those with whom we had limited contact and intervention. We were blindsided.

Without warning, Julia said to the group, "I just want you all to know how grateful I am that the CISM team called me when I was hurting so much about losing my best friend. When Marie died, I was suicidal. I wanted to kill myself. I did not want to be here anymore without her. I could not live without my best friend. I had a gun, and I knew how to use it."

"But then Colonel Jones called me, and I felt for the first time that somebody out there really cared if I lived or died. I told her I was not suicidal, but until she called, I was. If it wasn't for this CISM team, I wouldn't be here."

Julia could no longer email or talk to her friend, so at my suggestion, Julia wrote one last letter to Marie. She wanted to share that letter with the group. She read the following:

Dear Marie,

The time has come where I have to say goodbye because you gave your life while in the process of trying to save the life of another. I never thought that this day would happen because we were so close. I always hoped that I would die first so that I didn't have to feel the intense pain that I am feeling right now.

You were my best friend and I loved you very much. You gave me joy whenever we spent time together, and when we talked on the telephone. I always enjoyed eating out with you because it was the only time that we ever got to spend any time together (alone).

When we went to the SAREX in July, you and I shared a hotel room, and I asked you after we were on our way home if you still liked me even after we spent two days living together and you said yes. It was the most fun that I had ever had with you. We were like sisters, and I loved you very much. I will never forget the time that I told your dad that you liked sumo wrestling and the time that Moose (Marie's dog) kissed me. I hope that now you are in heaven with Joe and your mother and that you will remember me and wait for me with eager anticipation until I am able to join you in Heaven.

My heart will never mend. It hurts so much now that I feel like it is being crushed within my chest by someone with a strong hand. I wish that I could have been in that plane with you so that I could have died with you. You were all that I really had.

You made my day every time we got together or talked on the phone. I enjoyed all of your e-mails, and I read the last one that you sent me last night. I could tell that you were speaking to me through the screen and that you were saying that you loved me. If I could change things I would not have let you fly in that plane, but I know that you would have gone anyway.

You were really my hero because you loved me just like I am; you said that you didn't see anything wrong with me. I always questioned you because I was worried that you were just putting up with me and just telling me what I wanted to hear. You always told me not to worry; that we would always be friends and that there was nothing that I could do to change that.

I can't believe that you are gone. There is a big hole in my heart where you once were. My life was wonderful because of your friendship.

I joined the (volunteer disaster relief group) because I wanted to do more with you. You kept encouraging me to join even though I told you many times that I was not really interested. Thank you for the years of friendship that you gave to me. It will be a time that I will never forget. I was always thinking of you and wondering how you were doing and if we were going to get together soon.

I will never forget how much you gave me. You gave me unconditional love and a once in a lifetime friendship that not many people can say that they had. You made my life worth living every day just because you loved me.

I am looking forward to the day when I can join you in heaven and spend the rest of eternity with you. Thank you again for your friendship. I love you.

Following a heartfelt confession in debriefings, other participants will often share at a similar depth and intensity, and one can almost palpate the emotion in the room. There is also a sense of the initiation of healing, between the tears and laughter, by those who have loved and lost someone close to them. Debriefing participants learn the steps they need to begin that healing.

They have comforted and shared with one another. They receive referrals if the need is greater than a peer support system can provide. We assure them that we will be checking in with them in the days to come to make sure they are ok. We wrapped up Julia's debriefing, and the folks stepped out of the formality of our circle, dispersing to have cookies and punch, and visit with one another, and us, in a more informal gathering.

The CISM team met in a closed room away from the other folks, utilizing Dennis Potter and Paul LaBerteaux's method of Post Action Staff Support (PASS). PASS is a technique used to guide the discussion of the CISM team members to minimize any negative responses they may take with them, providing a way to transition out of the emotional demands of the debriefing. Debriefers sometimes have a tendency to carry away the pain of the individuals they've been dealing with (taking the job home with them), so we want to ensure that CISM team members stay strong, and are ready to go out again to help others.

Our team also discussed what went well, things we might have done better during the debriefing, where we stumbled, and what we might have done differently. The time came where we discussed Julia's confession, how impacting that was for all involved (CISM team members as well as the group that was being debriefed), and how no one had anticipated Julia's admission. After an extended period of intense and soundless staring while each of us searched inwardly for something to say about the possibility of suicide in the group we had just debriefed, Patty, the team leader, broke the concentrated silence by declaring softly but quite passionately, "A life was saved." A simple statement. Although the sanctity of the debriefing prevents discussing what happens in them, this is one example of why the ICISF (International Critical Incident Stress Foundation) model of debriefing works.

We followed the ICISF model and saw positive, life changing, and in this case *life-saving*, results. Had we not become involved, we would have been addressing a very complicated issue: three line of duty deaths *and* a suicide that followed because of improper crisis management. In that thankfully hypothetical situation, I would not have wanted to be one of the command staff involved in asserting that "no one needed" our interventions, to carry the guilt in knowing that they, by preventing the simple act of conversation, could have saved or cost a life.

Julia did what many of us do when we have a life-changing event. She went inside herself to heal and find answers. It was not a conscious effort (it rarely is), but the world kept going on as though nothing had changed. Julia saw it as a superficial wash over a painful emotional landscape.

Certainly, the world *knew* that it was a different place. When Marie died, there was a rift in the universe. A black hole formed, sucking into it the future that Julia anticipated along with hoped-for experiences and laughter.

Marie taught Julia so many things. She had value not only to Marie but also to those around her. Julia was part of the world, and it was an OK place to live sometimes. Not always filled with pain and rejection, tomorrow was more than another 24 hours of purgatory. While Marie taught Julia to live, what Julia had not ever fathomed was the lesson and legacy Marie would give through dying.

Although the movie *What Dreams May Come* (1998, Robin Williams and Cuba Gooding, Jr.) may not reflect the beliefs of the masses, it held a theory of the afterlife that gave Julia peace. The tagline of the movie was, "After life, there is more. The end is just the beginning."

Those words opened a door to new understanding that death is not necessarily an end. The body dies, but the spirit lives on. The essence of the person who sheds their physical cocoon continues, and sometimes visits us … in dreams.

Julia had one of those visits in her dreams. She was joyous at the experience of being able to talk to, and hug, her dear friend and emotionally adopted sister. Julia wrote,

Dear Sherry,

I finally got to tell Marie last night that I missed her and that I loved her. I had a dream about her where we met in a very bright room. I did not see anything else in the room but Marie.

I walked up to her with a little hesitation because I was not sure that it was actually her. When I got to her, I put my arms around her and held her close and told her how much I have been missing her, and she told me that she missed me too. Then I told her that I loved her, and she told me that she loved me too. Tomorrow is the first anniversary of her death, and I am finally able to face it with the knowledge that she is safe where she is and that I will see her again.

I talked to Julia yesterday. She calls to let me know how she is faring and sends emails to stay in touch. Julia is doing much better, healing and becoming as whole as she possibly can. She wanted me to know that she finally took the scanner training (as Marie had always urged her to do) and found it exhilarating.

With both feet set firmly on a path to continue in her volunteer work, Julia is seeing how important and fulfilling it is to concentrate on helping others instead of looking at her pain and loss. She clearly sees a greater value in her life and contribution to humanity through these works. Julia never rode in an aircraft with Marie, but even now while sitting in the back seat of a Cessna as part of an aircrew, Julia still looks up to Marie. She knows Marie is still looking down to guide her.

~~~

Sometimes the reaction to a critical event can remain buried for many years. Eventually, most of those suppressed items surface with a bang. This story is about one such experience. A medical professional was transformed in a way that she had certainly not anticipated, when she least expected it, in a way over which she had no conscious control.

Life passes so quickly that you do not always have time to stand back, assess, and digest information. Sometimes things happen so quickly that they slip under the radar of rational thought, going straight to your heart. Then you evaluate the emotional tugging after it knocks you off your feet, and you simply cannot stand.

Delayed Reaction

Working in the cardiology module of the ER, Nurse Carol* was oblivious to anything but the six acutely ill patients she was assigned for her shift. The sickest and most medically needy were usually the least demanding. The *walkie-talkies,* those who could and should have waited for an appointment to go to their family doctors, loudly and consistently demanded service throughout their stays.

It is funny how someone who has not eaten "in three days" is suddenly acutely hungry the minute he or she gets into an ER bed. A fresh pillow and blanket, and a real meal, please, not a turkey sandwich, cookie, and cup of juice, far outweigh medical folks' priorities. EKGs, blood work, IVs, and medications are secondary to creature comforts.

Carol did her best to keep up with the ungodly and unreasonable demands. As per usual, she skipped her lunch break and longed for a free moment to empty her bladder. Caught off guard and feeling completely overwhelmed, she heard The Scream.

The Scream is a sound known to pre-hospital and ER personnel. It is the guttural wail that emits from the depth of a fragile soul when they learn that their loved one has died. The Scream is unmistakable, and regardless what the ER staff is doing at the time they hear it, even if they keep moving physically, their hearts skip a beat. They might hold their breath, become nauseated, or experience goose bumps up their arms and to the tops of their heads.

They are all, no matter how tough, affected by that sound. The internal experience worsens when the staff is part of the team acting in response to the scream, to bear some accountability for the outcome of medical efforts. Hearing the scream from a distance is easier. The workers give each other a knowing look, take a deep breath, and get back to their world away from The Screamer's pain.

Carol could have done that—knowing look, deep breath, walk away—because resuscitation (the "Resus" module) was not her assignment that day. Something about the helper personality and mentality told her that she needed to respond. She left the safety of her adult population and answered that inner call.

She stepped out into the hallway in front of the ambulance bay. Perhaps Carol thought that she would just look, and someone else would come along to take action. She walked out just in time for a mother to drop a bloody three-year-old child into Carol's arms.

Carol tells me that she could not hear anything after that. She can still see the sidelong glance of the open eyes of the child. She can still see the blood. She does not know if the child was a boy or girl, black or white, and she was not sure if the child was breathing.

The walls and floor blended into gradations of gray and white, with irregularly formed streaks representing the auras left behind by the people who moved in slow motion around her. Turning on her left foot and leaning to the right, Carol somehow managed to turn her body and put her feet one in front of the other to make the forty-foot trek to Resus.

People began to gather as Carol stood holding the bloody child. She did not set him down, did not know what to do, and simply stood at the front of the four-gurney room. Resus gleamed with bright lights and stainless steel, a room efficiently lined with specialized equipment and towers of supplies used in resuscitative efforts toward making the impossible possible.

The charge nurse sat at the desk in the far corner of the room and watched, not moving, as the staff flooded into the room and prepared to treat the baby. Ten years of EMS and several years of nursing were lost to Carol at that moment. She could not think of what to do except to lay the child on the hospital stretcher and back away. Those assigned to Resus stepped forward and started working on the child, cutting away clothing, connecting to a monitor, and starting an IV. The child must have been alive because Carol remembers that no one was doing chest compressions or bagging, which they would have done if the child had been in cardiac and respiratory arrest.

Carol backed out of the module and went to the bathroom to wash the blood off her arms, scrubbing them for a very long time. She felt no matter how hard she scoured, she could not clean the blood completely off her hands and arms. Carol finally changed into a new set of scrubs brought by an ER tech who noticed Carol's scrubs covered in blood. She went back into her assigned module, finished her 12-hour shift, and then without a word to anyone, went home. She never asked, on that day or any other, about the outcome of the child dropped so unceremoniously into her arms by a mother looking for a miracle.

The next day was supposed to be fun. Carol and her boyfriend planned a day of flying gliders; a special treat because Carol had never flown in a towed and engineless airplane before. She had not slept, so when her beau, Kevin*, showed up at her front door, Carol was quiet and a bit withdrawn. Carol tried to ignore the fatigue. She decided to try to stave off the funk she was experiencing, and make the best of the day for Kevin's sake if not her own.

There was little conversation along the way. Carol, normally bright, articulate, finding any excuse for experiencing or eliciting laughter, could not complete a thought or a sentence. Kevin probably wrote it off to some *girl thing*, which was fine as he felt some things, like a long country drive, are not for conversation.

They went to the airport. It was surrounded by acres of agriculture as far as the eye could see, dressed with a lush grassy field and gently rolling hills. There were plenty of pilots gathered around the picnic table placed near the hangar, socializing and exchanging airplane talk. Carol wanted no part of it.

She excused herself, declined flights and refreshments, and went off to walk in the woods. Staring for a long time at the surroundings Carol was looking for answers, looking for something to make sense of the uneasiness she bore. She found nothing soothing in the trees or the clouds or the aircraft circling above. There was a rising anxiety in her gut that she could not explain.

Remembering the video camera at her side, Carol took photos of the planes as they took off, separated from their towlines, and landed. She remained a good distance from the other folks, who carried on with nonsensical conversations that she did not have the energy to pursue. Carol killed most of the day looking for tranquility in nature. For the first time, it simply was not there.

The clouds were not fluffy, soft shapes one could imagine as animals, faces, buildings, or trees. They were bloody clothing cut from a child's small frame, a vacant stare in an injured child's eyes, a limp body floating by. Instead of feeling shocked at seeing those reminders in every tree and plant around her, Carol felt numb. She was determined to keep walking farther away, trying to escape herself, to outrun the anxiety that continued to grow.

There was a tree in the wooded area lining the grassy landing strip that Carol remembered staring at for a very long time. She photographed the tree so she would never forget its shape. She says it looked like a mother with a large empty womb in the center, lonely, old, and barren. Dying. Her heart ached empathetically for the tree and its loneliness.

At the end of the day, Carol climbed into the car with Kevin, and they stopped for fast food. Kevin playfully taunted Carol with a few French fries, which elicited only revulsion and nausea. Kevin pitched the fries and stopped for pizza, thinking that might help, but it did not. Carol could not eat, and awake for almost two days, found her thinking becoming more bizarre.

As much as she did not want to admit it, that child's vacant, staring eyes still haunted her, and she was not sure she had gotten all the blood off her arms. Carol felt removed from herself, watching her life with a clinical distance, as if it belonged to someone else. Physically, she began feeling an all-over sense of tingling, as if a phone set to vibrate was going off somewhere on her person, but there was no phone. Carol stared at her arms looking for spots of blood she may have missed.

When Kevin escorted Carol safely inside her home, she asked him to stay, telling him that she was afraid to be alone, and not entirely sure why. Kevin laughed uncomfortably at her, declining the invitation and saying that he had to meet with a client early in the morning on the other side of town. Carol was almost in a panic about being by herself.

She feared another sleepless, dark night seeing those eyes staring to the side, and that small body covered in blood. She did not tell Kevin about the patient or her feelings. Someone outside of the medical world would not have the capacity to understand, much less offer a way out of the darkness.

Carol sat upright in the center of her couch as Kevin closed the door. She tried to gain control of that unidentifiable something that had her in its clenches for more hours than she cared to give. The situation and her emotions neared subdued hysteria. Carol thought to herself, "Come on, old girl... this is crazy. *You are* crazy, or you are going to be. *What is so different about this child?*"

Carol had a long time to think and finally, somehow, the answer came to her. She was not mourning *this* child; she remembered *her* child. Somewhere in the depths of her heart and mind, Carol finally allowed the long-buried memory to surface that she had lost her baby

20 years before, almost to the day. An unborn child never named, very much loved, and very painfully lost.

In the twenty years that passed, Carol worked hard at suppressing the memory and the pain. She stopped panicking at the anniversary date, thinking at some point in those years that she was *over it*. Nothing could have been further from the truth.

As with any buried or suppressed pain and trauma, eventually, the censored memories come bursting to the surface. It takes a lot of energy to keep abnormal normalcy's in place, and that three-year-old patient covered in blood tore down every last wall that kept Carol safe from her grief. She finally had to face it, mourn the loss she never allowed herself to acknowledge openly or grieve, and move on.

There is never an easy solution or painless way to care for old, deep wounds. Carol's approach to dealing with the situation and her pain was to accept that the circumstances surrounding her baby's death were something beyond her jurisdiction. Instead of keeping it a secret that no one else knew, except her apathetic ex-husband who considered the unborn child disposable, Carol started talking.

The more she talked, the more her experience changed from a nightmare to a memory, eventually becoming something she could lay to rest. She shared her pain with those who understood with their hearts as well as their intellect. She will never forget, but Carol found that sharing her story and her loss with others in similar circumstances gave her a way to offer comfort and understanding to those who felt alone in their pain. She feels it is the best way to honor the child. To honor both children; the one who died, and the one she hopes survived.

~~~

Hurricane Katrina devastated countless people in so many ways. However, for some of the rescuers, the experience was life-changing in a positive way. One national Critical Incident Stress Management (CISM) team working with a paramilitary group found an opportunity to reframe the workers' experience and let them walk away feeling like heroes.

These boots on the ground troops focused on constructive contributions instead of losses. They had a positive impact on the people of Mississippi, and each other, in their travels to and from the work site, and while performing their duties. This story shares some facts of the disaster: The strategic planning of those who came to help, the good some took away, and most importantly, the hope.

Katrina: After the Storm

On Monday 29 September 2005, Hurricane Katrina hit the Gulf coast of Mississippi with full force. Katrina was one of the five deadliest hurricanes in the history of the United States. The two-day path of destruction through Mississippi hit all counties, rendering them a disaster area, and affecting more than one million people.

Many areas suffered injury by the storm's wide path. Damage in outer bands included tornadoes spawned by the hurricane. As a paramilitary group working with the United States Air Force, our team was deployed to Jackson, MS, and three forward operating bases (FOBs) for disaster and crisis response.

The Mississippi Emergency Management Agency (MEMA), by way of the US Coast Guard (USCG), tasked Civil Air Patrol to perform three missions. 1) Make contact with USCG personnel who had not reported in after the storm. 2) Support MEMA missions as assigned. 3) Provide support for the 1st Air Force and outside agency missions.

While CAP trains and practices for actual missions and exercises, nothing could have prepared them for Katrina's challenges. The IC (Incident Commander) of the mission was CAP Maj. Owen Younger. Captain Younger prepared and delivered a stunningly intuitive response plan in the worst of circumstances.

Strategies include setting up phone lines, computers, printers, and Internet connections. Communications occur through cell phones, with equipment in air-conditioned rooms. Typically, these operations centers are far from the billeting, galley, and *off-time* areas of response teams.

In the aftermath of Katrina, those commonly accepted amenities and tools were unavailable. The billeting, galley, and operations center were often in the same room (or tent). Standard expected amenities, such as running or drinkable water, air conditioning, equipment to warm food, and a daily shower, were fond memories for the first responding teams.

CAP's ground mission during Katrina was to make contact with individuals in four counties at the southern tip of the state. The mission headquarters (HQ) in Jackson, MS was supported by three forward staging areas: 1) Stennis AFB, 2) Wiggins, and 3) Pascagoula. "The operational concept," per Younger, "was to attempt contact with individuals on a residence-by-residence basis in areas where contact would be most beneficial to the people remaining in those areas, and then to perform short interviews... to identify any needs." The Air Mission was multi-dimensional, utilizing aircraft's digital imagery "for the state and federal needs, for transport of critical personnel (both CAP and other), for lifesaving flights, for direct resupply of ground teams, and for airborne communications platforms," said Younger.

With the magnitude of the disaster and number of troops arriving for disaster response activities, it was no wonder that CAP CISM would be included to support responders potentially traumatized by rescue efforts. Around the country, many CISM teams anxiously awaited deployment, as did the CAP CISM teams, pending word from the appropriate CAP/USAF channels. After more than 10 years of organizational development and team growth, there was an active CAP CISM team, a plan in place for deployment, and a national CISM Director who's 'A' team was packed and ready to go before the winds hit category three.

The adventure had begun, the plot line was in place, but much to the frustration of the CAP CISM team members, there was no order to deploy. Attempts by the CISM Director to talk to the mission IC and either of the top two in the national chain of command, Maj. Gen. Antonio J. Pineda, or Brig. Gen. Rex Glasgow, failed. We could not communicate with the command staff through satellite phones, radios, or cell phones, so while operations at the four bases continued, there was no CISM intervention the first several days.

We, as CISM team organizers, worked closely with our sole contact for the disaster, Deputy Director of Operations (National Headquarters) John W. Desmarais, Sr. (a.k.a "Moose"). Moose and I had become close friends during many years of collaboration while working to develop CISM in CAP and this was our biggest challenge to date. We were in touch every couple of hours those first days while waiting for the "Go" to set people in motion to put boots on the ground in Mississippi. God bless Moose, who kept Don Brown and me in our seats while we waited for official permission to set our plan into action.

It was astoundingly difficult to wait for the order to "Go." Moose kept us from self-deploying, which would have been a grievous error. In CISM, if you are not invited, you do not go; we waited rather impatiently. Some folks did not adhere to that universal directive.

Away from the disaster site, with communications intact and television broadcasts supplying endless updates on the devastation, the CAP CISM team members around the country wondered why they were not called into action. As coordinators of the CAP CISM teams we, Lt. Col. Sherry Jones, and Chaplain Lt. Col. Don Brown relayed information and made tentative travel arrangements. We prepared the first crew, first relief, staff rotation, and for the next hit. Hurricane Rita was on the horizon, which Chaplain Brown lovingly called "Marga-Rita," noting that by the time Rita fully hit the Gulf Shores, a Margarita would be welcomed.

We knew that for deployment purposes, we were restricted to two CISM team members per base. Limited to eight souls to send into our war zone, those painstakingly hand-selected and eminently qualified CISM team members readied to book flights, and prepare ground vehicles, to get to the disaster area. Their fully self-sustainable ready-gear contained uniforms, supplies, bedding, water, and foodstuffs. All eight reported their availability of boots on the ground within 24 hours of *Go*.

They stood by their phones waiting for a phone call from Don Brown or myself to give that order. National CISM Staff Members, Administrative Officer Capt. Christopher Latocki, and Maj. Paul Brown, Information Technology Officer, were already preparing for follow up to the first deployment. The CISM National Deputy Director Lt. Col. Don Brown would stay home to run the team and prepare for rotations while Lt. Col. Jones, coming in from Detroit, led the team to the site.

It was a painful decision for Lt. Col. Brown to stay at home when he wanted nothing more than to be in the thick of the disaster response site. However, he realized that there were only two people in the country with the ability to lead the national team. One had to go to the disaster site, and one had to lead from home. Lt. Col. (Dr) Joan Coughlin came in from Massachusetts to provide crisis intervention and mental health supervision for the disaster site HQ and forward operating base teams.

Responding to the situation and not following a textbook written-in-Jell-O plan of action the CISM coordinators disposed of Plan "A." In actual disaster response, teams often throw out the initial strategic plan. I repeatedly hit redial to Gen. Glasgow's cell phone, until the wee hours one morning, when the General happened to be standing in the right place at the right time, and the airwaves allowed a call to go through.

General Glasgow told me that two chaplains had come to the HQ site, and finding no request for their training specialties, pulled CISM certificates out of their bags saying, "Well, then we can do *this*." The General and administrative staff thought these two men had been deployed by the national CAP CISM team (they had not). Therefore, the NOC (National Operations Center) did not deploy the real team. With those delays set aside and later appropriately handled, the General and I resolved the issue. The real team of eight CISM interventionists (four peers and four mental health professionals) deployed and were boots on the ground within 24 hours of the order to "Go" as promised.

When we reached Jackson, Mississippi, we barely had time to drop our bags before stepping into a briefing with the IC (Incident Commander). The CISM team members and crews for the three forward operating bases received their orders and flew immediately to their sites. Sat Phones (satellite phones) and radio contact were sporadic and ineffectual.

We often lost signals in the middle of conversations, so we knew that our initial planning meeting with Maj Younger could be the last time we spoke until the team reunited a week later; it was. Members like Maj. Paul Brown relied on training and instincts to perform their duties in the face of unanticipated challenges. My gratitude to Maj. Brown continues, for his actions during those challenges and prayerful support afterward.

Our four teams were each comprised of one male and one female, combining one mental health professional and one experienced multi-credentialed peer member. The exception to the male/female pairing was at the headquarters, with Dr. Joan and me as the female/female team. Like so many other disaster-relief volunteers around the country, we left our jobs for the week and carried everything with us that we would need: bedrolls, food, water, and all ancillary supplies, including toilet paper.

Some of us had access to showers and some did not. In anticipation of deployment, I cut 14" off my bum-length hair knowing that I would be in a military uniform and unable to shower for a week. It seemed appropriate at the time, but my husband made me promise never to do that again.

Dr. Joan and I were at the HQ site at the request of the National Commander. The General wanted "the best" and most experienced pair for the Command Staff, and those who were stopping at Jackson before release home. When we reported to the hangar in Jackson, we received strange glances from staffers who were unsure of our duty assignments. People did not know what CISM teams could do at a disaster site.

We quickly made friends and proved ourselves useful assisting the HQ staff with small duties, like tallying up fuel receipts, and giving shoulder rubs while discreetly performing our CISM duties. I am not a trained massage therapist, but what little we covered in nursing school came in handy. I would highly recommend having a massage therapist with a chair for emergency services workers as it provided stress relief for our folks.

During each massage, a casual conversation (one-on-one intervention) permitted speaking directly with each member of the command staff. We tried to ease their burdens even if only slightly. Tensions were high.

The command and headquarters staff tried to meet the needs of the client, keep their troops responding, and planes in the air. They attempted to ensure that all troops had food, water, and fuel. They hoped that each got adequate rest and down time and that there would be appropriate warm bodies for rotations at the end of the outgoing troops' duty week.

Fuel, scarce and difficult to obtain, was a major concern for those who drove several hundred miles to get to the mission headquarters or forward operating bases. Katrina was a completely new ball game, and those at ground zero stressed about calculating needs and arranging response teams. Those who were at home waiting for deployment did not understand the delay, and almost all were at peak frustration even before beginning disaster response duties.

Eventually, power returned to our mission HQ home, the hangar, which also became a clearing center for supplies. Contributors who made their way through the damaged roadways dropped canned goods, coffee, paper supplies, packaged dried fruits, desserts, powdered milk, MREs, and bottled water. Heavenly provisions indeed, and using the kitchenette in the hangar, we kept a pot of coffee going for troops that stopped by or worked at the HQ. Those donated provisions meant ensuring our pilots and ground crews had fruit, albeit canned, for the week. It also gave us an opportunity to speak with those who passed through Jackson at the beginning of their duty assignment, or before they headed home.

The mental health professional overseeing the operation, Maj Joan Coughlin, PsyD (CAP National Clinical Director), shed her "Dr" title as well as her gold oak leaves. Our office door reflected that change, and humor, reading: "Auntie Joan: *The Doctor* is IN." Pilots were especially hesitant to share feelings, so Joan found a clever way to approach them.

Food was an issue, and most members were subsisting on MREs (military Meals Ready to Eat), so when foodstuffs were dropped off at the mission HQ, Joan found a case of individual servings of applesauce. She sat down with each of the aircrew members between sorties (flight duty assignments) and asked, "When was the last time you had some fruit?" Proffering the applesauce, even the toughest among them would soften, graciously accept the offering, and cautiously pour their hearts out. Dr. Coughlin became, "Auntie Joan, the Applesauce Lady."

Discretion *is* the better part of valor, and our CISM team members were those unsung heroes who never expected thanks or recognition. Paul Brown, assigned to FOB Wiggins, Mississippi, was my on-site spiritual rock and remains a prayerful friend. Each team member brought specific and special talents to the disaster site that made them invaluable. Like the rest of the disaster-relief workers, they lived under the stars with a smile on their faces, ready to do anything asked of them.

Billeting was a challenge for Auntie Joan and me, as there were no provisions in the hangar for females. HQ had an all-male staff. Because three stars (two generals) requested our presence, a tiny room became the place to put our bedrolls. It was cramped and smelly, but we were grateful for a roof over our heads instead of bunking under the stars with critters.

We slept in a standard small office with a large metal desk and bookcase. The furniture was too heavy to move. Joan slept behind the desk, and I slept in front of it, with my head in front of the door, and our legs curved around the side of the desk. There was not enough room to stretch out even though we are both barely 5'4" tall.

We joked about playing footsies for the week, reminding ourselves that we were away from critters and vermin. The floor, carpeted many years before showed the wear and tear of countless pairs of boots, smelled like a musty combination of AV gas (aviation fuel), dust, and dirt. We did not spend much time sleeping, so we were practically unconscious during those few hours we spent on the floor.

On our final two nights, we received folding cots to get up off the carpet. Unfortunately, we found that the cots did not have enough room to unfold completely. We spread our bedrolls over the accordion bumps, another point of humor to our situation, and yet another moment that would find absurdity in later storytelling.

The male officers at HQ had it a little better. They shared one large room where they spread out their bedrolls, sleeping bags, and cots. The pilots stretched out in the communications room (sleeping three), and the command staff had the more private commander's offices, with a couch.

As a former midnight nurse on an interventional cardiology unit, I can tell you that a room full of snoring men is not ideal. Joan and I considered our shared semi-private room lush accommodations. Because it was *my* head in front of the door (which opened inwards), I was fortunate that no one entered without knocking. If a medical or CISM emergency occurred during the night, each person had the courtesy to knock and announce himself before attempting to enter and risk denting my head.

The CISM team had planned, in pre-deployment discussions, to provide demobilizations and one-on-one interventions. CAP practices these ICISF model interventions, built into regulation as the CAPR 60-5. We thought we would be giving general information to off-going or end of duty day troops. We planned to have personal conversations with the ground troops, aircrews, and command staff.

What we found were people greatly in need of much more. We quickly re-strategized to provide on-scene support services while filling each day with one-on-one conversations and defusings (small group discussions) for each team as they prepared to return home. In this circumstance, it was mandated by the command staff and ordered by the IC (Incident Commander), and the Maj General, that *all* staff would participate in the interventions proffered by the CISM team.

Operations staff at a mission site lists the day's activities on a dry-erase board. The exact CISM intervention was not pre-determined until the assessments of each day, and each situation, were made, so the term *Outbriefing,* provided by Captain Eric Hudzinski, was coined and used. It meant that each troop had to report to the CISM team before releasing from duty. This gave the CISM team leader the option of how they wanted to manage the Crisis Intervention portion of the mission appropriately.

Micromanaging by untrained people who do not understand CISM is never wise. Credit and kudos go to the two generals in this mission who wisely not only left the planning to the experts but also ordered the participation of all members. These officers (the CAP National Commander and Vice Commander) participated in a defusing before leaving the duty area themselves. Strong leaders always lead by example; Generals Pineda and Glasgow did so for CAP CISM.

The mission participants did not have to talk, but they *did* have to sit down with the CISM team before releasing from duty. The benefit to all was clearly apparent, and many who had initially shunned the group discussion later expressed their appreciation. One very experienced ES Officer said it was the highlight of his trip (to Jackson, MS). He gave me his unit patch, which I still treasure.

CAP's participation in Hurricane Katrina reported, by the end of the mission, the participation of 214 individuals. They exceeded 14,615 man-hours and included 19 echelons of personnel from 16 states. Ground team, aircrew, and mission base staff worked a 6-7 day rotation to prevent excessive fatigue.

The CISM folks at the HQ base were the first ones up in the morning and the last to sleep at night. We made ourselves available to individuals who wanted to talk when no one else was around. Quarters were very close, limiting privacy.

We successfully defused every ground crew who stopped at the HQ building before they left to travel home. We used the male quarters, the largest room in the back of the hangar, for our group discussions. The room afforded privacy and an opportunity for us to walk the members through their experiences. We provided education to normalize their experiences, address their concerns, and ensure they had someone to talk to when they got home. We did not ask, "Do you have someone to talk to" but "*Who* do you have at home to talk to," which included family pets.

We let the troops know we would be available to them after they left the headquarters, and that someone would be calling to follow up with them. We gave them a contact number to call if they needed us before we called them. In the defusings, whose specifics remain private, a theme emerged that we had not anticipated.

The theme was similar to 9-11 and many other disasters. The rescuers/ES workers were frustrated at what they perceived to be a delayed deployment, and at not being able to do more. We could help those who responded to the Katrina disaster to understand not only that had they gotten there sooner they could not have gotten through, but also that there was nothing more for them to do across the boundary road. Everyone and everything on the other side of that road was dead.

The National Commander commented later that even from the air at 2,000 feet above ground, the stench of death was unmistakable. We managed to turn the troops' expectations and experiences around to a positive note, one which some communicate to us even today as having been helpful in understanding an experience and situation that defied explanation. Instead of walking away feeling as though they had failed by not doing enough, they left with pride at what they had accomplished in their tour of duty at Katrina.

During their disaster-relief duties, some of the ground teams had unexpected experiences when they approached homes to take a census and to assess for the immediate or emergent need of the inhabitants. As they asked if the folks needed food, water, or medical care, the workers were stunned to find time and again that the *victims* offered whatever little they had to share with our ground troops. One family cooked their last chicken and offered the troops, who carried and shared MREs, part of their last meal. As the CAP ground teams passed out bottles of water, many residents asked if the troops had enough water, as they wore full field gear in that Mississippi heat and humidity.

More than one gas station attendant refused payment when the troops stopped to fuel their vehicles. More than one party store gave the troops free snacks when they stopped, appreciating that the teams had come from as far as the Northeast region of the United States. The craziness that occurred after Katrina garnered national press and attention. Not every one of our experiences was so positive, but much needs to be said for the spirit and sense of community and humanity held by the folks in Jackson, Pascagoula, Stennis, and Wiggins, Mississippi.

Regarding CISM support, Katrina's mission IC, Owen Younger, wrote:

> This mission brought with it considerable stress factors which, combined with long mission base duty hours and somewhat primitive sleeping arrangements, after a time began to impact the effectiveness of all personnel on the mission. The effect of these

factors on a mission of this magnitude is both expected and inevitable, but with CISM support, this impact was alleviated to a great extent.

When Maj Younger rotated out, the IC replacing him, Lt Col Rickey Oeth, wrote:

> It has been previously stated that the CAP CISM team played an important role assisting members with coping with the inevitable stresses and strain this kind of mission will produce. In any future operations of this kind, CISM teams should continue to play a part, as their value is felt long after the event is over.

The former method of coping with this and lesser levels of stress was to 'hit the bar' for a time of conversation and drinking. Sometimes this coping strategy lasted well into the night and with far too much alcohol consumed. As Chaplain Lt Col Don Brown is fond of saying, "Alcohol doesn't drown your sorrows, it just teaches them to swim."

> Even though it got off to a rocky start, having a CISM plan in place made an enormous difference to the CAP members. As with all actual disasters, many lessons learned add to best practices for future endeavors. Members of the USAF auxiliary organization recently, at the anniversary marking of Katrina's mission response, remembered the positive things that came out of their service. In many cases, CISM interventions helped to turn attitudes around. Troops moved from anger and frustration to satisfaction for a job well done. They recognized the value of assisting those with tremendous losses in a positive way. (Maj Younger)

When I got back to Detroit Metropolitan Airport after the mission, still in Battle Dress Uniform (BDUs), I was exhausted. I did not remember where I parked my car. I tearfully called my husband to assist in thinking through the process of finding it.

Walking from the gate to baggage claim was incredible. My CISM team members had a similar response from airports around the country as they traveled home: gratitude. People stopped us and said, "Did you just get back from Katrina?" As we replied that we had, people's eyes softened, some tearful, as they said, simply, "Thank you. Thank you for whatever you did."

We felt invisible until those moments, and rightly so. We do our work privately and silently. We do not tell with whom we spoke or what happened during those conversations. However, we carry with us the pride and fulfillment of knowing that in many lives, we have had the opportunity to make a tremendous difference.

We provide a transition between Hell and home after a disaster situation. It lets the worker move from thinking about what they could not do, to seeing what they *did* accomplish. They realize how much they *did* help. For those who carry painful memories, we help them in learning how to get back to the lives they left.

Receiving recognition was surprising and humbling. I wanted to tell them I was the one who received help. I was the one who grew. I was the one who had a different view of life and a greater understanding and appreciation for all the blessings I had been given. Exhausted, all I could think to say was, "You're welcome."

I dropped my bags off at the front door of my home, grabbed a quick shower, and headed north to see my mom. The closest significantly large city to Mama's home was about 50 miles from her, so I always stopped there to get mom a Big Boy fish sandwich. I was shocked to stand in the restaurant and look around as I waited for her order.

There was fresh water given to the patrons as they sat down at the tables, whether they wanted it or not. There was food everywhere, in great supply, and everyone was clean and dressed in comfortable civilian clothing. Looking outside, the buildings were all intact, the landscaping impeccably groomed, with cheerful red blooming flowers surrounded by lush greenery.

After only a week on a disaster site, I had forgotten what the real world looked like, how plentiful supplies were, how we so easily took the basics of life for granted. As I drove the rest of the trip north to Mama's home, I was numb. I expected to cry, but it still did not seem real. Tears would wait.

Katrina affected all who were involved in many different ways; some very painfully, some with great loss and sadness. I think my team and I can look back with great pride and appreciation for having had the opportunity to provide a positive impact. We shared a humbling duty of being without creature comforts and family for a short time, of making comparatively small sacrifices. We gained far more than we gave, and to this day, we remain close because of Katrina.

For that, I am eternally grateful.

In Remembrance, Rex E. Glasgow
January 1, 1959 - December 9, 2016

Writing has become a method of dealing with inner conflicts. It helps to understand and resolve issues that confound me, a self-help home therapy. I write (or more accurately, I type), I disentangle, I move forward.

In CISM courses, we often tell folks to journal their feelings while working through the emotional aftermath of a traumatic incident. Give no thought to penmanship, syntax, spelling, sentence construction, or content. Just let the words and ideas flow; write until you feel exhausted, then write some more. Penmanship changes as you break down the walls of control and get to the internal 'good stuff'.

If you cannot write, use a voice recorder, and when your voice changes, that is when truth emerges. Do not read what you have written for two weeks. Then go back, read, and respond in writing to what you have written. Very revealing.

My daughter, Missy, took a college creative writing class. She had to delve deeply into her own inner mental and emotional sanctum. The journey revealed to her, and to me, feelings she did not know existed. Missy gave me permission to share some of those thoughts and her emotional response to a traumatic situation.

What Did You Do At Work Today, Mommy?

Over the years, I have made many references to my children in essays. You write what you know, and I know my babies. In this book, I wrote about Missy's desire to be in emergency medicine since she was eight years old. Her essay corrects me; she says she was seven, and she is right. So much for the precision of parental memory.

Our combined memories about a particular incident, however, are a little more accurate. They tell of the pain encountered when Missy finally began following in her mother's footsteps to work in emergency medical services. It rather reminds me of an adage: Be careful what you ask for because you just might get it. Missy writes:

As far back as I can remember I wanted to work with patients. When I was a child, my mother was a paramedic; it was at that time in my life, at the tender age of seven, that I decided I wanted to do what she did. Every day I would ask her how she saved lives and the details that came with the task. 'What did you do at work today, Mommy? Did you save anybody's life or see anything gross?' My favorite question was always about what she saw ...

What did I tell her? Surely, I minimized the pain and suffering endured by the patients and glamorized the rescues to make the stories more exciting. Increasing the drama helped portray her Mumma as the hero.

Storytelling communicated the elation I felt working in such a phenomenal profession. Having someone rapt with interest and awe at the accomplishments of the day fed us both. Missy listened intently, egging me on to tell more stories, so eager to hear every detail of each shift.

We spent hours together poring over medical books showing normal anatomy, and what happens to the human body through illness and injury. Missy was transfixed with each tale and every picture. Most kids never wanted to see that sort of thing, but my little one could not get enough. Missy dove into the books herself and was never repelled.

In later years, she introduced me to online sources of actual photographs of trauma found through her continued search and thirst for understanding. I could not keep that child out of the books, and the questions she posed were intelligent and intuitive. She had a natural talent and understanding of all things medical. She maintained that she wanted to be able to do everything I did without ever attending college.

She was a smart child, but there was a bit of a handicap that soured her on formal education. Her brother's IQ was upwards of 170. Missy always felt like the odd man out when the three of us got rolling in some heady discussions that flew over her head with an almost audible *whoosh*.

Missy did not lack intelligence. She is a very bright young woman, with more common sense than her brother and I combined. The legacy of having a genius brother can be intimidating, though intimidation was never her brother's intent.

Quite the contrary, he too loved to teach and share wonders with the little sister that he adored. Although he was nine years her senior, they learned from one another. Eventually, they became my teachers as they matured and developed personally and professionally. Missy writes:

> I wasn't the normal child that found blood and guts disgusting. I was the child that wanted to see the pictures and hear the gruesome stories every day. I would look through [my mother's] textbooks just to see what could happen to the human body in trauma and medical situations. I loved every picture and

story so much that on the day that I graduated high school, I understood my destiny.

I enrolled in an EMT course and in 10 weeks, I was a certified Emergency Medical Technician. Two short weeks later, I was employed at St. Jean Hospital and Medical Center* in the Emergency Room. That is where my life changed forever.

When Missy was 15, she shadowed me on a midnight shift in the emergency room. *Take your daughter to work day* takes on new meaning in the ER. We took extensive steps to assure ER management that Missy was mature enough to handle what she might see.

Agreement to let Missy work a shift with me came only after I contracted to keep her out of the resuscitation module, where all the bad stuff happens. Later, as an employee, Resus was the place she came to work more often than most other techs because she excels at functioning at that level of expertise and demand.

We worked the Ortho-Trauma module that night, a section of the 75-bed trauma center treating mostly orthopedic injuries, and probably the least emotionally traumatizing. Unfortunately, triage placed the combative and inebriated patients in trauma module, too. Missy did not bat an eye at restrained patients who yelled the kind of things that children are not supposed to hear, showing an impressive level of fortitude for one so young and inexperienced.

During the night, Missy had the opportunity to assist me with a procedure. We were short-staffed, and I had to handle something normally done by two nurses. There was a woman with a dislocated jaw who needed conscious sedation and mandibular reduction. As the nurse, I inserted the IV, prepared the patient, gave the medications, and ensured that she continued breathing during the procedure.

Missy hit the buttons on the monitor and reported the patient's vital signs and any changes in her SPO^2 (oxygenation) every two minutes. Of course, the monitor was good at beeping whenever there were any abnormal numbers, but Missy did not know that at first. She took her job of assistant seriously, did not flinch at the procedure ("it was cool"), and finished out the night as one of the best assistants I had ever had. Three years later, Missy formally joined our ER family.

Missy is beyond comparison as the best tech I have ever worked with, and that is not Mom talking. This praise comes from a staff nurse who had a job to do and a sense of urgency to get it done. When you have unimaginable demands in the hospital, there is no mother-daughter preferential treatment, and there is no time for familial coddling. As an ER tech, Missy held her own, obeyed every request and direction without complaint, and never said a word about being up all night to work the entire 12-hour shift:

> *Beep! Beep! Beep!* My alarm was screaming. I peeled my eyes open and slapped my hand into the general direction of the annoying sound.
>
> The clock read 1:05 pm and I knew that I had run out of time to hit the snooze button. The previous night was my first 12-hour shift, and I was exhausted. Unfortunately, I had to wake up and do it all over again. What I did not know was this particular day was not going to be like any other day I had lived.

Welcome to the world of emergency services. Missy's shift would be 3 pm to 3 am, the worst hours of the day (and night). It is the most active, the highest volume, and the most traumas. When my daughter Missy jumps into something, it is with a round-off back handspring, lots of attitudes, and she nails it. She is her mother's child. Her orientation period was on the day shift with me, 0700-1930:

> As I was sitting in the break room at work, chewing on a disgusting cheeseburger that the cafeteria so graciously provided to us, I was rudely interrupted when the overhead paging system blared, 'Code One Trauma, ETA five minutes.'
>
> When [a code one trauma] is paged overhead, it means that there is a patient coming in that has been in a very traumatic accident or has an injury so bad that it might have to be fixed in the operating room. I excitedly swallowed the last bite of my burger and jumped from my seat. My first trauma code!
>
> Pushing open the trauma room doors I yelled, "What's coming in?" I was grinning from ear to ear. My hands were so sweaty I couldn't get the gloves on them.

Many newbies get excited at the thought of working a code, especially a trauma code. That level of challenge is indeed exhilarating, testing their developing skills and critical thinking abilities. Newbies know that they will finally have hands-on experience with what they have been learning about in books, and excitedly anticipate using those skills.

Knowledge and experience marry in a funny way. The information goes from the instructor or pages in a book into one's head and then has to find its way out through the student's hands in actual application. What often does not occur to the neophyte is that a patient is a real person. Sometimes the information does not go straight from the head through the hands but takes a detour through the heart and the gut. That moment of connection and gut reaction, when the worker personalizes the situation, can be problematic.

Missy continues with her story.

> 'Chill out Missy,' yelled Dave, my preceptor.
>
> 'Weren't you excited when you got to see your first trauma code' I asked.
>
> 'I've been doing this for 10 years. I have forgotten the feeling. Just get your gown and mask on; they will be here in 10 minutes.' Dave wasn't the happiest of people, but he was good at his job.
>
> A second later, the triage nurse burst through the door. She reported to the trauma team standing by, 'Gunshot wound to the head. No vital signs present. The call over the Bio-Com was broken up, and I couldn't hear the age of the patient.'

The triage nurse takes radio reports over the bio-com. Ambulances call in ahead of time when they can. Sometimes instead of being several minutes out they say, "We're at your back door." The purpose of the radio call is to give warning to staff so the ER might prepare with appropriate personnel for whatever EMS is bringing to them.

In Missy's hospital, the nurse takes the radio report, writes it down on a piece of paper, and takes that paper to the resuscitation module. She gives her verbal and written reports to the nurse in charge of the module. The doctor is included in that report when he is present. Then the nurse goes to the ambulance doors to clear the way for the incoming trauma.

Very often this effort includes emptying the hallways of equipment and rubber-neckers. Folks who hear the announcements of an incoming ambulance love to peek out into the hallway to see what is coming ('Just like on TV!'). In the case of a gunshot wound to the head, the likelihood of survival is already low. Even though there are tense moments, a trauma team knows what to do and mentally prepares for the situation.

Located at the outer edge of the murder capitol of the United States, this hospital got gunshot wounds (GSWs) almost daily. It was expected and rarely got anyone's adrenaline pumping. Codes were also a daily (or multiple times daily) expectation of the staff, usually handled without a lot of emotional response -- unless it was a child. Missy continues:

The most important piece of information is whether the patient has vital signs, which include heart rate, respirations, and blood pressure. If there aren't any vital signs present, the patient is dead. The age is the second most important piece of information. It tells the staff which doctors should be present and what equipment needs to be ready.

Not a moment later, Detroit EMS came barreling through the doors and rushing to the cart that held multiple trauma team members, staff physicians, and an eager 18-year-old girl that was trying to get her feet wet. What I saw next was the picture that hasn't left my mind all these years.

A 7-year-old boy was lying on the EMS, stretcher and the paramedic was doing compressions on his tiny chest, trying to bring back a heartbeat. We moved the boy over to our stretcher as the paramedic was giving us report with a troubled voice: 'This young man was with his cousin in the garage playing with his father's rifle when it went off.' After giving us that small piece of information, the paramedic quickly left the room with tears in his eyes.

The boy's vital signs still hadn't returned when our staff took over. We started giving multiple medications to try to revive his little body. My stomach turned every time that I looked down at him. He had been staring down at the large rifle when it discharged a bullet into the left side of his face. The doctors had called his time of death shortly after arrival.

Minutes later, it was time to prepare the body for the family to say their final goodbyes. I had to wrap the young boy's head so that his mother and father didn't have to see their child the way that I did.

Reading this now, I am somewhat angered. I first read this story when Missy had written it for a college writing course. However, through fatigue or perhaps the emotional protection of not understanding what I read, I did not comprehend, or want to comprehend, the most important fact. Missy is the one who prepared this boy's body.

She was 18 years old, straight out of high school, and newly into the job. Her preceptor should not have left her with that chore. It was unkind and unprofessional, or at the very least exhibited bad judgment. The preceptor should have walked her through preparing the body, instead of leaving her alone so he could smoke or hit the break room.

That is the problem with some emergency folks. They have no critical thinking skills. They say, "Let the newbies sink or swim. If you aren't tough enough then you shouldn't be here. Let us see what you are *really* made of! You have to prove yourselves to us, and only when we deem you worthy will we treat you as an equal."

Different coworkers expressed the thought that working EMS or ER is a divine dispensation. It is a privilege to work at this level of trauma. If the God of Emergency Medicine has not anointed you, you should find yourself a desk job or flip burgers.

We are the aristocracy of emergency services, the savers of lives, the keepers of souls, those with the power to save lives. Not everyone thinks like that, thankfully, but some make the transition from the outside world to ours harder than necessary. That attitude sets many people up for failure, since we are all, indeed, completely human.

I had to stop almost every minute to wipe the tears from my face. When I was finished applying the dressing to his wound, I walked into the staff room and buried my tear-stained face into the first person's chest that I saw.

I did not know what she had gone through. I was not the one there for her when she was in so much pain. I worked that day, was not far from her, but caught up in the craze of my module and patient demands. I did not even see her until later. As I ran from my module toward the lab with a handful of tubes containing blood I had drawn from a patient, she stopped me in the hall just in front of the Resuscitation module.

Breathlessly, she said, "Mom, do not go in there." Missy pointed to the Resus room, whose doors closed uncharacteristically at both entrances. "You don't want to see what is in there."

Missy's face lowered in a way I had seen many times since she was a child. It was not like her to cry when she was emotionally bothered or in pain. She was tough. To control her emotions, she looked down, holding in the tears and the complaints, focusing on the floor, or a place in her heart and mind where she felt safe.

I saw that face for the first time when she was three. I was going to the hospital to have a hysterectomy. I said I would call her from the hospital every day, several times a day. She was sitting in the back seat of the car, looking down, and said, "No, Mama. Don't call. It will make me miss you more. I'll see you when you get home."

I knew that there had been a GSW. The announcement rang overhead while I was starting an IV on the patient whose blood I carried when I met Missy in the hall. After I dropped the blood tubes off at the lab, I immediately did what Missy begged me not to do. I went into Resus to see what was so terrible that she wanted to protect me from seeing it, from feeling the pain she felt in its presence.

The boy was in bed three of Resuscitation. He was an African-American child, slight, and very attractive. He looked like he was sleeping. There was a white bandage carefully wrapped around his forehead hiding the horror that brought him to us.

His eyes finally closed, Missy had covered him in a crisp, white cotton sheet. I went to his bedside, although I have a particularly difficult time with pediatric patients. I had a pre-hire agreement not to work in the pediatric module. For 11 years, I stayed away from children as much as possible, though I had my share in Resus, which I could not avoid. I had to take a couple of deep breaths before lifting that carefully and heartbreakingly applied bandage.

Adept at slipping into an emotionally distancing clinical mode, I told myself that I had to see what everyone else had seen to understand Missy's feelings. I lifted that bandage. I saw several holes through the boy's skull, then peeked into the skull to see a depressed brain.

Clinically, it was very interesting, because I did not have any responsibility in the effort to save his life. Knowing that he was dead, and that I was simply examining a body, I was safe from the emotional effects. I forced that distance because I knew the next step would be to observe the rest of the trauma staff to see if they were as troubled as Missy was.

As I left the room, I saw Joe, a nurse with many more years of experience than I have in working this sort of trauma. I think he might have been the person who Missy grabbed for a moment of comfort when she tearfully went into the employee break room. Joe was Italian, which bonded us to him, and he worked on that little boy, linking Joe and Missy further in understanding what no one outside those doors could grasp.

Joe was coming out of the break room blowing his nose and wiping his eyes. I had never seen Joe so affected by a patient before. I asked if he was ok and he smiled and patted my arm, "Yeah, I'm fine."

From that point, I walked the 30 feet to the cardiac module and looked at my tech, Bill,* who had helped with the trauma. Sometimes people are not assigned to Resus will assist when patient resuscitation requires as many hands and warm bodies as will fit into the room. Bill had a handful of lab tubes, a tourniquet, a butterfly needle, two alcohol preps, some patient labels, and a roll of tape. Bill gathered those items in preparation to draw blood from a patient, but he was walking from the desk to the supply cart, back to the desk, and at one point walked literally into a wall.

His eyes were red and glassy. Bill made a few failed attempts at taking those supplies to the patient's bedside to draw blood. He looked at the labels, looked at the dry-erase board with the patient names to see what bed to go to, looked back at the labels, and again at the board.

I took the tubes from his hands. I said, "Bill, go to the break room and sit for a few minutes, or have a cigarette, or go for a short walk. Just get away for a little bit and I'll handle this."

I called the ER social worker and asked her to come to my module. "Liz,* are you going to have a crisis intervention for the staff for the GSW to the head of that seven-year-old?" Liz looked at me quizzically. "Why? Do you think they need it?"

I said, "Joe is a hardened veteran and not only is he is walking around in tears, but he has not been back to his module to work. Bill was just trying to draw blood from a patient and could not figure out how to do it, and I saw him walk into a wall. Missy has been crying and has a thousand-yard stare when I can get her to make eye contact. Yes, I think you need to do something."

Liz called the hospital crisis team and arranged for a defusing at the end of shift (1900h/7 p.m.). Those who wanted to talk could do so before going home. CISM interventions provide some level of closure to the workers, so they do not take the crisis and their responses to it home with them. The participants are given tools to deal with the aftermath of trauma when the code is called, and it isn't over for them, so the worker can lay the incident that shook them to their core finally to rest ... or at least begin the process of inner healing.

The worker receives assurance that he is not deficient or going crazy because the incident bothered them. They are human. Their responses are human and appropriate in the face of senseless tragedy.

I saw Missy in the hall. She was scheduled to go to her EMT class immediately after work. I asked her to stay for the defusing. "I can't. I have school, and I can't miss it."

I told her I thought it was important to attend the defusing. "You can do that for me after work tonight. You do it for everybody else all over the country, so you can sure as hell do it for me later."

Missy does not swear at her mom—ever. She was right. I was working CISM all over the United States for CAP. I taught crisis intervention. I ran the CAP National CISM Team. I flew to *Anywhere USA* to do debriefings with almost no notice several times a year.

Surely, I could do something for my daughter. Her response clearly demonstrated that the situation was not over with the end of the code. For many who worked on that child, it was far from over.

The social worker showed up at 1900, and those who could leave their modules attended the discussion. It was not the ideal situation, as the hospital really should have provided coverage for all who wanted to go to the meeting, pulling them out of service for a short time. The hospital did not make those arrangements.

It would have been better to have a peer experienced in ER to assist with the group discussion, validating the social worker, and providing the *I've been there* point of view. I stayed after my shift and stood outside the door of the room where they held the defusing. It was happening within the ER, again not ideal, since anyone could have come knocking on the door, save for the fact that I would not let that happen.

It only took about 30 minutes before the door opened and the group dispersed, some to go home, some to go back to their modules. Shifts overlapped, and Joe was working 11 a.m. to 11 p.m. I asked Joe if he was ok, telling him that I could stay for the rest of his shift, or cover for him until he was ready. I was off the clock, so I was available.

He smiled that winning Italian smile, looked like he was back in his skin, and said he would be ok for the last four hours. The other staff members who walked out of the room also looked a little more lucid, seeming somewhat relaxed and more at peace. I made a mental note to talk to them a little later, since one meeting is not enough, and although the social worker said her door was open to them if they needed it, no one would come back to her. It is not in the ER mentality to ask for help, although talking among ourselves is acceptable.

When Missy was growing up, I worried about her. ER/EMS moms are more knowledgeable about what can go wrong, knowing the horrors that most folks never have to consider. She was an athlete, and pretty tough, but even though her brother watched over and protected her, Missy seemed to take the things that go bump in the night a little harder. I tried to keep them both safe and failed miserably more than once.

When Missy was a child, I heard a song that touched on the relationships and wishes I had for both of my children and Missy remembers me singing it to her... a lot. It was Billy Joel's Lullaby, "Goodnight My Angel," which seemed fitting since I had always called my daughter Missy Angel. I wanted the kids to know that if anything ever happened to me, I would always be with them. They had only to close their eyes, and I would be there for the rest of their lives.

Missy married a firefighter paramedic named Scott and continued in the lifestyle she dreamed about. She is in her second decade with the same hospital system and has become a veteran, but not like the one who told her to chill out because he did not get excited over trauma codes anymore. That guy burned out and left, which happens too many times to those who work ER for too many years. It takes its toll.

Missy is also more realistic now. She knows that it is a rare instance when we bring the dead back to life, but hope survives knowing that those days do occasionally happen. She has become predictably hardened to those who abuse the system or the staff, but still has an incredibly tender heart, especially for children and older folks. I admire her.

I asked Missy to think about the difference between now and then. Think about her perspective surrounding the call that shook her to her foundation, and the way her preceptor delegated the child's body care. She replies:

> Now I would look at [the dead child] as just another patient. Would I have put another 18-year-old in that situation to do what I did? No... but they wanted to see if I would sink or swim. I've seen many more dead babies and children since then, and you just keep going or become a receptionist.
>
> I think the [crisis management] help offered there (at the hospital) is a joke. Some stranger sitting there alone with us asking, "How do you feel?" doesn't work. It would have been more helpful to talk to someone who has done what I have done instead of a stranger who hasn't had that experience and is just asking me questions.

I asked her several more questions. "Do you think having that type of response to a patient could happen to you again?"

> Probably. The last time it happened to me was 2-3 years ago in Resus when I had five people die in my shift, the last patient of the day was my age, and he died of a drug overdose. I just couldn't take any more; too much for one day.

"Do you think you know the type of situation that would be difficult for you to handle, even with years of Trauma Center experience?"

The one thing that would put me—or anyone—over the edge is child abuse. That is something nobody can handle, and we get more than you would think; nothing dramatic, nothing causing death, but I've seen (them) badly injured.

"Do you still like what you do?"

I'm getting ready to get out; I'm about done. Everyone asks me if I'm going to nursing school, but I tell them I don't want to do this anymore. I don't think there is anything I haven't seen.

You come to a point where you've just seen enough. Burnout; your head is full of the memories and the faces of those you worked on that died. If I sat and thought about it I could sit and see every patient I've ever had; all those faces stick in my head as I'm sure they do in yours.

Scott had a call the other day that blew his whole day ... a 16-month-old baby with multiple medical problems who had a seizure in his mom's car. Scott had to tube the baby in the car seat, upside down. He delivered the baby to the hospital after working so hard to keep him alive, and the doctor ripped out the tube and tried to re-intubate the baby because there was air leaking around the tube.

The doc couldn't get the new tube in, so the baby coded. Scott was so frustrated because he fought so hard to keep the kid alive only to have someone undo his work. The baby lived, but we don't know how much damage was done.

I'm thinking about doing business management or health care administration, but no more direct patient care. I love taking care of people and being there (in the ER), but I started so young that I've had enough. I don't want to lose the ability to take care of my own family.

I'm paranoid now (about the unseen dangers that no one else realizes exist), and our children are going to be screwed. One parent from the ER, one from the road, and a grandmother who has done both. Our son will have to live in a bubble.

Missy eventually left the trauma center for a smaller ER, then moved into a clinic. The emergencies are more manageable, and as the lead medical assistant, she has some level of control. Her son wants to grow up to be a firefighter paramedic. Missy and I are hoping he will opt for something like a plastic surgeon.

~~~

This story and others came from the perspectives of innocence, and from experience. Some were traumatizing and others were completely exhilarating. There has been laughter, lunacy, and sometimes, a hint of lasciviousness. In all cases, though, they are my life and echo the type of situations emergency services workers around the world face every day, and with similar outcomes.

We share the joy and insanity of working in the streets or the ERs. Until our last breaths, it will be part of who we are. Our jobs define us; they motivate us, and they sometimes cause us to run away from ourselves, even though we take ourselves wherever we go.

I have tried to share with you stories of hope and redemption, showing that beyond the unexpected and painful circumstances there is a brighter place. With eyes wide open, we see a new landscape punctuated by pearls of wisdom, a new life and perspective awash with new and hopefully clearer understanding. With the guidance of our older brothers and sisters, we are less naive, we are calmer and more accepting, and we have learned not to sweat the small stuff.

We sometimes cry when children die, especially so needlessly and brutally as the boy who touched Missy's heart. Then we go home, hug our children, make popcorn, and watch a movie (happy endings only, please). We tuck those we love into bed and have semi-restful sleep that prepares us for the next day, the next go-round with death, dying, grief, and loss. We cry when a patient reminds us of someone we love, or of ourselves. Although we try to give every patient excellent care, whether we identify with them or not, there are those that end up on our prayer list at night because they got just a little closer to our hearts.

It does not begin or end with me. Things have changed dramatically since I started in Emergency Services, both in emergency medicine and paramilitary rescue. We have come so far in refining our rescue tools, abilities, and training.

Old school thinkers who live in a different reality, who feel you are tough, or you are not, do not always accept newer methods of coping. Some rescuers still fall through the cracks and do not receive the help they need when deeply and emotionally affected by their work. The legacy lives on.

New faces and hearts join our world, enthusiastically beginning their walk every day with a deep passion for helping those in need, to make a difference in this world, in the lives of those around them. Some of their expectations are rooted in logic and are doable. Some are sheer fantasy. They can lead newbies down a road to disappointment and disillusionment, to personal harm, and loss to the worker if he does not know how to get out of the emotional abyss that sits in wait.

Whether dealing with fact or fancy, the newbies' hearts are usually in the right place. We need to watch over them, to help if the puddle they step into becomes a raging river. One can only tread water alone for so long before succumbing to fatigue.

We do the things that people should not have to do, see the things people should not have to see. If we have not done so already, we need to learn a healthier way to do our jobs, to stay removed enough that we accept death as a part of life. For many of us, too many times, at the end of the call, it is not really over.

~~~

About the Author

Where did you grow up?

I was born in Detroit and raised in its suburbs, living with and around economically and socially challenged populations most of my life. There is a unique perception of the world when you grow up poor. Fortunately, being a second generation Italian-American, the ethical influences of my parents and grandparents taught appreciation for what you have, self-accountability, patriotism, and pride. The Midwest taught me a sense of community, caring, and connecting with your neighbor, leading to the desire to save him.

Why you are uniquely qualified to write this book

I can tell these stories because I have lived them. Like many, I grew up watching EMS and ER shows on television, and they seemed to focus on the hero aspect with predictable outcomes. While the television and movie representations are more true to life these days, there are still thousands of untold stories. My slant is in telling the side of the story you may never know about.

My stories tell how the emergency services worker feels about his experience. They reveal how the occupational trauma affects him, sometimes for the rest of his life. They share what he is thinking as he is going through the calls, and how he internalizes most of the bad thoughts and experiences. They reveal what happens after the call is over.

Why did you write this book?

Whenever I tell people what I do, they are immediately interested in what I have seen. They want to know about the gory side of life that draws people and prevents them from looking away. What they do not realize, until it happens to them, is that those horrible experiences happen to someone who is loved and cherished, especially the children.

I want people to see the world, for a moment, through my eyes. I want them to walk with me through the broken glass, to sit next to me and hold the hand of the injured or dying. I want them to know, for a moment, about our constant fight against death. Then I want them to see the complete lunacy of it all and laugh.

What do you think readers will get out of it?

I am hoping that readers will see emergency service workers in a new light, and realize we are human, too. We have our challenges, pains, and sorrows. We have surgeries and broken bones. We have been in accidents, and our backs are killing us from lifting. We have sick kids at home, and would much rather be with them than earning a paycheck, but we have responsibilities.

The misperception I get almost daily in the ER is that "you don't understand what I'm going through." Maybe not, but you might be surprised. Because we hold our tongues during work hours, maybe some readers will appreciate knowing what we are thinking. This book shares what some of us ponder when we leave our professionalism at work, strip off the uniform, and settle into an easy chair at home.

What will you do next in your life?

Back in school full-time, I am working on a post-surname alphabet soup. With a master's degree in psychology, specializing in crisis management and response, I am in the final stages of a doctorate in education. In crisis management, your experiences only carry you so far; the academic world says you have no voice without a terminal degree. Yours truly is tweaking that voice.

When I wrote the first edition of this book, my laundry list of to-do items included co-writing with a dear friend, George W. Doherty. I missed that opportunity. I miss George even more. The checklist changes but never seems to get any shorter.

The priority: spending more time with family, especially the grandsons. Plans include more books, collaborations, and branching out into related areas. Returning to CISM training, developing more workshops, especially for nurses, and reinvesting in trauma response is likely.

Or maybe I will just become a crazy cat lady.

~~~

Glossary

#10 Can: An aluminum food storage container that holds about 14 cups. Think big ol' can o' coffee.

Achilles heel: A weakness or vulnerability.

ACLS: Advanced Cardiac Life Support; established protocols for advanced medical care of the patient who is having a serious medical emergency, which includes resuscitation.

Adrenaline: A naturally occurring "fight or flight" hormone, it is also a medication used in resuscitative efforts (epinephrine) to treat cardiac arrest or arrhythmias (abnormal electrical activity in the heart).

Advance Directive: A legal document that outlines the patient's wishes if he is in a position where he cannot verbalize them himself (as with severe illness or injury).

Algorithm: A sequence of instructions used to carry out a specific procedural plan of action aimed at a goal of care or resuscitation; the plan has a definite ending point.

Annie (doll): CPR (Cardio Pulmonary Resuscitation) mannequin used for training purposes.

Antecubital (vein): The vein found in the arm in front of the elbow.

Asystole: No cardiac electrical activity; no heartbeat.

Ativan: A benzodiazepine drug used to treat anxiety (anxiolytic: "anxiety breaker") or as a sedative to calm, relax or tranquilize.

Atropine: A medication used to speed up the heart if too slow (bradycardia) and in cardiac resuscitation efforts.

Autistic: An impairment of the growth and development of the brain demonstrated by difficulties in social interaction and communication inclusive of repetitive behaviors, often manifested in early childhood.

B-52: A combination of two medications, Haldol 5mg and Ativan 2mg (B for "Bomber" and 52 for the amount of Haldol and Ativan given, respectively, in milligrams). Haldol is an antipsychotic medication.

Bag Valve Mask (BVM): A handheld flexible bag with a reservoir (for oxygen) and tubing leading to an oxygen tank, its mask is held to the patient's face and bag manually compressed to ventilate a patient (may also connect directly to an ET or endotracheal tube); also known as an Ambu bag.

Bagging: The process of compressing the Ambu bag to ventilate a patient.

Barium: A liquid given to a patient orally or via enema for a clearer view of certain organs when x-rayed (internally absorbed).

Bio-com: Radio communications between agencies, such as a hospital ER and ambulances or area dispatchers.

Bipolar: A mood disorder often characterized by swings between mania (abnormally elevated or irritable) and depression, formerly known as manic depression.

"Bodies... The Exhibition": The controversial exhibit of preserved cadavers shown in various stages of dissection displayed in different collections of poses. Several exhibits travel around the country to show the internal workings of the human body.

Buck up: Slang term meaning to grin and bear it, to not be affected by the circumstances around you, to "get over it.'

BUN: Blood Urea Nitrogen, a blood test that measures renal (kidney) function.

Cannulate: To insert a tube into the body.

CAP: Civil Air Patrol, United States Air Force Auxiliary.

Cardiac arrhythmias: Abnormal heart rhythms.

Cardiac monitor: A device that shows and prints physical tracings representing the electrical activity of the heart.

Catheterization: A medical procedure whereby a tube is inserted into various body parts for diagnostic or treatment purposes.

CC's: Cubic centimeters, a measurement of volume used by the medical community to designate volume of dosages.

Cervical: Of or about the neck.

Chuck Hole: The hinged 4"X12" slot in segregation cell doors.

CISM: Critical Incident Stress Management is a comprehensive, integrative, multicomponent crisis intervention system. This system's approach underscores the importance of using multiple interventions combined in such a manner as to yield maximum impact to achieve the goal of crisis stabilization and symptom mitigation. (Everly and Mitchell).

CO: Corrections Officer (not guard); a law enforcement agent who participates in the containment, custody, and security of prisoners, themselves, and corrections staff, mainly in jails or prisons.

Code: A code usually refers to CPR in progress. Someone who loses pulses and respirations codes. If coding an ambulance, the vehicle is traveling with lights and sirens.

Code status: Medical care facility (or EMS) term referring to the procedures that can be performed on a person who suffers cardiac or respiratory arrest.

Compressions: The accepted method of responding to cardiac arrest by externally pressing on the chest/heart to move blood throughout the body (when properly performed by trained rescuers in resuscitative efforts).

Conscious sedation: A hospital administered process whereby medications produce an altered state of consciousness allowing the performance of medical procedures.

Control / Control Center: The functional nerve center of a corrections facility, Control coordinates communications and is responsible for internal and external security.

Creatinine: Chemical waste from muscle metabolism, which is filtered by the kidneys and excreted in the urine.

Crepitation: The sound made by bone ends rubbing together **D-card:** The designation given by a particular company to identify the ambulance call (the dispatch number).

Cutting/Cutters: Cutting is non-suicidal self-injury or mutilation, usually with a sharp implement on the skin, which can reflect an underlying psychiatric problem. Cutters are those who self-harm to feel better, a method of dealing with negative emotions like rage, guilt, emptiness, self-loathing, etc.

Delusions of grandeur: A psychopathological condition whereby the person has irrational or inappropriate fantasies of power, wealth, position, or omnipotence (supremacy).

Dextrose: Glucose; sugar in the body for energy or in medical applications, can be given through an IV as a treatment for things such as low blood sugar.

Diaphoretic: Profuse perspiration, covered with sweat.

Drug box: A box usually made of lightweight but rugged plastic that contains emergency medications inclusive of strong narcotics, carried and used by Advanced Life Support paramedics in the field.

Dry Stun: Pressing a Taser directly against the flesh and delivering an electric shock without deploying the prongs.

Dump: When the patient suddenly takes a turn for the worse, possibly into an irreversible situation such as death.

Ecstasy: A synthetic stimulant street drug that gives effects such as exhilaration and produces an increased sense of intimacy with others as well as a decreased sense of fear and anxiety.

EMT: Emergency Medical Technician, or 'Basic' EMT.

EMTI: Emergency Medical Technician-Intermediate, sometimes known as EMT Specialist, is a mid-level provider with more advanced skills than a basic.

EMTP: Emergency Medical Technician-Paramedic, a highly skilled EMT with training in Advanced Cardiac Life Support and other advanced lifesaving techniques; may administer some medications.

Endotracheal tube: (ET Tube) A tube that is inserted into the airway of a patient into the lungs to allow ventilations; the tube is inserted in-hospital commonly for general anesthesia and in pre-hospital patients who cannot breathe on their own.

Epiglottis: A tiny flap of tissue that sits at the end of the tongue and covers the trachea when a patient swallows, allowing food to proceed down the esophagus into the stomach instead of entering the trachea (windpipe).

Epiglottitis: An inflammation of the epiglottis that is a true medical emergency, as the inflamed flap can completely close off the airway causing death if not treated promptly and aggressively.

Epinephrine: A medication used in the treatment of cardiac arrest and certain arrhythmias and anaphylaxis (acute severe allergic reaction).

ES/Emergency Services: A collective term for organizations that work in several aspects of public safety, disaster response and preparedness, etc.

Euphoria: Intense happiness and well-being sometimes obtained through chemical means or in a psychoaffective disorder.

Faces of Death: An explicit film series showing graphic dismemberment and violent acts from the late 1970's, they show a collection of death scenes from multiple sources.

Flatline: The physical tracing on a cardiac monitor that shows no electrical activity of the heart (a flat line) that occurs in cardiac arrest.

Foley catheter: A tube inserted through the urethra into the bladder to drain and contain urine.

Fugue: In a dissociative (mind distancing) fugue, a person flees their home and surroundings to get away from whatever major stressor they experienced.

Full arrest: Complete cardiac and pulmonary standstill; no heartbeat, no breathing.

Golden Hour: The 60 minutes immediately following traumatic injury in which treatment is most effective to increase chances of survival.

Gown up: Putting on personal protective equipment and attire to prevent bodily fluid exposure, such as a surgical gown, gloves, booties (foot protection), goggles, and face shields.

Gumby Suit: The anti-suicide gown is a heavily quilted one-piece sans collar or sleeves, and too thick to roll and use as a noose.

Gurney: A wheeled stretcher or hospital cart (upon which patients lie).

Haldol: (Haloperidol) An antipsychotic medication used to calm patients who are in an acute psychotic state, delirium, or mania.

High flow: An oxygen delivery system that gives patients the highest possible concentration of oxygen through a mask; 'high flow' means turn it all the way up.

HIPAA: A privacy rule for patients stating that confidential information will not be released to anyone without the patient's consent and protects individual's insurance coverage when they change (or lose) jobs. It stands for Health Insurance Portability and Accountability Act (of 1996).

Homeostasis: The body's ability to maintain a balance, to regulate itself to remain stable.

Homicidal Ideations: Thoughts of harming another person.

Humerus: The long bone in the upper arm (shoulder to elbow).

Hyperventilation: To breathe or cause someone (through ventilations) to breathe very rapidly.

Ibuprofen: A nonsteroidal anti-inflammatory medication used to treat pain and inflammation.

Identity crisis: An inner conflict where a person is not sure who they are or their role in life.

Impotent: A man's inability to attain or maintain an erection.

Incarceritis: Any acute illness erupting upon arrest or incarceration in a healthy individual; usually resolves upon placement in an ER bed.

Insectivore: A creature whose diet consists mainly of insects.

Intubate: The process of placing an endotracheal tube in a person to allow them to breathe.

Joe Medic: The slang term given to paramedics (usually newly in the profession) who have all of the toys, bells, whistles, and markings (on their homes, cars, and clothing) noting their profession. They are defined by their jobs.

Jonesing: The slang term for a strong craving or desire for something.

Jugular vein: Vein(s) in the neck that drains blood from the head to the heart.

Jump kit: The bag a paramedic carries with all of his lifesaving equipment.

Jump seat: The seat directly behind the driver that faces the stretcher in an ambulance patient compartment (back of the ambulance); it is where the medic who is caring for the patient often sits.

LEO: Law Enforcement Officers, keepers of the peace.

Ligated: A medical term meaning to tie off with a suture (stitch).

Lobar: Having to do with a rounded anatomical part of the body, in this case, the brain (there are also sections of lung called lobes).

Maalox: An over the counter anti-acid medication thought to have magical properties, used to treat various and sundry ailments in the prison system when inmates become enraged unless they receive medical treatment from the nursing staff.

Mandelbrot set: Named after Benoit Mandelbrot, a set of points in the complex plane, the boundary forms a fractal, a geometric shape that splits into parts. Son Topher understands them; I just think they are pretty.

Mandibular reduction: A medical procedure done under conscious sedation whereby the dislocated jaw (wide-open mouth) goes back into place, and the mouth can close.

Manic: A phase in Bipolar disorder when the patient is possibly hyperactive, self-centered, euphoric, sometimes has unrealistic fantasies, and schemes, sometimes exhibits irritation or rage.

MAST pants: Military Anti-Shock Trousers formerly used by EMTs for stabilization of fractures or providing pressure to the lower extremities to move the blood up to the vital organs in the body.

Medical complaint: The reason the patient is seeking medical attention and treatment.

Medical control authority: A state-assigned group that is responsible for overseeing the emergency medical services in whatever designated area is named (such as a county or counties).

Medically cleared: No discernible medical cause for the patient's current situation (complaint) and they are ready to be evaluated by a psychiatrist or psychiatric social worker.

MoM: Milk of Magnesia, another over the counter medication widely used by nurses in the prison system for inmates complaints of constipation.

Ml's: A unit of measure that stands for milliliter, one thousandth of a liter.

Morphine: A narcotic pain reliever.

Murphy's Law: An adage that states if anything can go wrong, it will.

Muzzle Loading: Sticking things in the urethra (penis)

Nauseated: To feel sick in the stomach, possibly to have the desire to vomit.

Newbie: A slang term designating someone who is new to the profession and lacks the experience and knowledge of a veteran, a newcomer.

Nitroglycerine: A medication given for heart conditions, the desired effect is to open the blood vessels around the heart to increase blood flow and oxygenation, thus reducing or eliminating pain.

Observer (ES): A member of the small aircraft flight crew who sits next to the pilot in the front of the aircraft and has complex and specific duties assisting the pilot in air search and rescue operations.

OPlan: Plan of action for an emergency services operation.

Oral airway: A small plastic device placed into the mouth by medical staff that keeps the tongue from occluding the airway, also known as OPA or Oropharyngeal airway.

Packaged: Prepared for transport utilizing whatever tools are necessary to stabilize the patient in anticipation of ground or air transport to a medical facility.

Paddles/leads: The medical equipment that when placed on the patient's chest gives a reading of the electrical activity of the heart. While both will give a cardiac tracing, only the paddles have the ability to relay a shock.

Peer support: People with similar backgrounds or experience that provide emotional and practical assistance to those who have been through a traumatic situation.

Personal Protective Device: see PPD

Peter Principle: A management theory stating that people rise to the level of their incompetence.

Plato's Cave: An allegory describing the experience of people, chained to a wall viewing shadows of things out of view that becomes their reality and speaks to the effect of education.

Porter: Inmates with the assigned and respected responsibility of cleaning; they may receive a stipend and extra privileges.

Potassium: A naturally occurring mineral in the body that can affect kidney and heart function.

PPD: Personal Protective Device is a small plastic rectangular gizmo the size of a garage door opener with a clip on one side that attaches to corrections' staffs' clothing. In an emergency, the staff member will pull the string hanging from the top of the PPD, a light in the prison Control Center will indicate location, and several big strong folks with weapons

will respond to save the aforementioned staff. Theoretically.

PRK: Photorefractive Keratotomy is a laser eye surgery designed to correct nearsightedness, farsightedness, or astigmatism by changing the shape of the cornea (eye surface).

Prognosis: A prediction of medical outcome.

Prostatic: Relating to the prostate gland found only in males, which stores and secretes a clear fluid, and evaluated by a physician during a rectal exam.

Psychotic: A psychological condition whereby there is a break with shared reality; the patient may see or hear things that are not apparent to anyone around him and exhibit bizarre behavior.

Pulse Oximeter: A device used to measure the oxygen carrying capacity of the patient's hemoglobin (oxygen saturation). It is non-invasive, usually a device that attaches to the patient's finger or ear, also gives a reading of the patient's heart rate.

Pulse: Discernible and palpable heartbeat found by feeling the patient's arterial pulse points (such as at the wrist, the neck or the groin).

Regurgitate: To throw up, vomit.

Rescuer personality: A stereotypical characterization of the kind of people who work in emergency services fields such as Police, EMS, ERs, Firefighters and disaster relief occupations.

Ride along: A program whereby unlicensed personnel accompany professionals to become acquainted with the roles and responsibilities of those professions. In EMS, the person riding along (or third rider) may be in training but has not received certification or licensure to perform their duties independently, but may do so under licensed supervision.

Rig: Slang name for the ambulance; also known as a truck.

Risk stratification: The method of assessing a patient's history and complaint to determine whether they warrant immediate and emergent care.

Rounding: The process of walking through the medical area to review the patient's complaints, care, test results and status; usually performed at the change of shift between off-going and on-coming staff.

Rubber-Neckers: A slang term used to describe people who crane their necks to view the scene of an accident or some other situation that is usually morbid in nature.

Run Report: The written report made by EMS workers detailing the patient information, treatment, and outcomes.

Saline lock: An IV line inserted to give venous access, closed off at the outer end instead of connecting to fluids or medications.

Sally Port: A series of doors or gates that secure a passageway between points used in places like prisons or entries to secure inpatient mental facilities.

SAREX: Search and Rescue Exercise.

Scanner (ES): The trained flight crewmember in an air search and rescue operation sits in the back seat of the small aircraft, visually scans the area, and locates the desired search object (as in missing person or debris of a downed plane).

Schizophrenic: Person who is not experiencing a shared reality and experience with those around him (inclusive of such things as delusions or hallucinations); a psychological disorder.

Shanks: Also known as Shiv, any bladed device (knife)

SICU: Surgical Intensive Care Unit.

Sinus tachycardia: A cardiac rhythm whereby the heart is beating faster than normal, usually at a rate of greater than 100 beats per minute.

Snow (the patient): Administering medications to give the patient sedation and an altered level of consciousness; too much can depress respirations and cause the patient to stop breathing.

Spike lines: The process of inserting a sharp spike (connected to tubing) into bags of IV fluid to prepare them for patient administration.

Spilling cookies: Throwing up, regurgitating, or vomiting (also known as tossing your cookies, spewing, and puking).

Squadron: The military (or paramilitary) designation for a group of people at the lower end of a larger command structure above a flight, and below a group.

Stroke: Term for a CVA or cerebral vascular accident—a brain attack—from such things as a clot (denying oxygen) or bleeding in the brain.

Suicidal ideations: Thoughts of self-harm, includes the desire to take one's life.

Suppressing: The usually unhealthy process of pushing thoughts and emotions out of immediate awareness and trying to ignore rising emotions and unpleasant facts.

Ten-code: The established method of communication used by police, which gives numbers to represent certain phrases: 10-4 means okay, or acknowledgment of the previous verbal communication.

Therapeutic Conversation: A specialized method of conversation usually utilized in medical or mental health situations whereby the discussion may have a more positive outcome.

Tones: The sounds emitted through pagers and radios, usually from a central dispatch authority, that are specific to the desired responding unit and instruct them to react (normally to some emergency).

Toradol: (Ketorolac) A non-steroidal anti-inflammatory medication used for moderate to severe pain control.

Transport: The process of moving a patient to a medical care facility or from one facility to another either by ground or by air.

Trauma armor: (A way of) arming people in high-risk occupational groups and whom are at high risk for things like acute and post-traumatic stress disorder... to arm them with a sense of "psychological body armor" so that they become more resilient to trauma and stress factors.

Trauma Junkie: The slang term denoting someone addicted to the acts of responding to and assisting with medical trauma such as codes, car wrecks, and seemingly impossible rescue situations. Also, see, "Sherry Jones."

Tube: The slang term for an endotracheal tube, or ET, the tube inserted into the patient's airway into the lungs to allow ventilations.

Umbilicus: Belly button, the depression in the middle of the abdomen.

Urethral culture: A swab inserted into the penis to gather cells for analysis, usually when suspecting a sexually transmitted disease.

Vagal out: A medical term indicating a neurogenic vasovagal episode, also known as fainting.

Venous: Through the vein; blood that is returning to the heart.

Ventilation: The act of moving air through the lungs by natural or artificial means, as in breathing, bagging or placing the patient on a ventilator.

Vital signs: The measurements of respirations (breathing), blood pressure, pulse, and temperature taken by medical professionals to assess body functions.

Wingspan (human): The measurement from fingertip to fingertip when the arms spread out to the side of the body.

The World: Outside the locked doors and layers of barbed wire where people, non-inmates, live and roam freely.

Writ: A written order directing prison to deliver an inmate to court.

Yankaur: A specific type of oral suctioning tool used to remove secretions from the patient's mouth, the tube has a large opening on the end.

Index

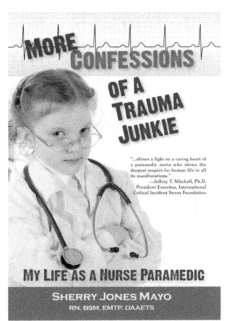

"...shines a light on a caring heart of a paramedic nurse who shows the deepest respect for human life in all its manifestations."
—Jeffrey T. Mitchell, Ph.D.
President Emeritus, International Critical Incident Stress Foundation

MY LIFE AS A NURSE PARAMEDIC

SHERRY JONES MAYO
RN, BSM, EMTP, DAAETS

More True Stories from EMS and the ER

More Confessions shares the raw and honest feelings of emergency service professionals through true 'story behind the story' revelations. Disclosing experiences from both sides of the gurney, Sherry and other EMS, ER, paramilitary, and firefighter responders walk you along their fragile line of sanity. Using humor as a life raft during perfect storms, workers reflect upon how they endure and survive personal and professional tragedy while trying not to care too much, and what happens when they fail in that attempt. A graduate student in psychology, Sherry is a paramedic, trauma nurse, and crisis interventionist who led a national paramilitary crisis response team and continues conducting crisis management training throughout the U.S.

Emergency Service Professionals Praise *More Confessions*

"Once again, Sherry brings to life the overlooked or, too often, over-hyped world of the emergency services for all to experience. She does so with a vitality and spirit that makes her prose almost poetic. If you want to glimpse the amazing world of EMS from 'behind the curtain,' *More Confessions* is for you. Highest recommendations."
—Rev. Don Brown, B.A., M.Div., Flight Paramedic (retired), Chaplain, Lt. Col., CAP (retired); Pastor, First United Methodist Church, Grand Saline, TX

"*More Confessions* will take you to the edge of first responder insanity with honesty and integrity. Sherry has once again opened our world to the reader by cleverly describing the unbelievable experiences that we have every day. This book is the real deal!"
—Peter Volkmann, MSW, EMT, Chief-Stockport NY Police Dept.

From Modern History Press
ISBN 978-1-61599-141-9